wheat & gluten free

JODY VASSALLO

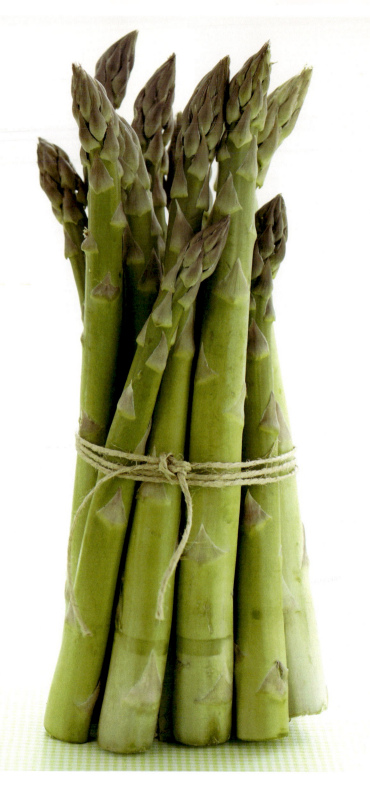

GLUTEN-FREE EATING

Most frequently it is people who suffer from coeliac (pronounced 'seeliac') disease who require a gluten-free diet. Those with the skin condition dermatitis herpetiformis also need to eat gluten-free foods. It is estimated that coeliac disease affects 1 in 260 Caucasians worldwide. Dermatitis herpetiformis is much rarer and is usually seen in people who also have coeliac disease.

Gluten is a protein found in large quantities in wheat, triticale, rye and barley, and, to a much lesser degree, in oats. Ingredients derived from these grains may also contain very small amounts of gluten. Avoiding gluten removes fundamental foods such as wheat bread, pasta, biscuits, cakes and pastries from the diet. When wheat products are baked or heated, the gluten sets, leaving an aerated, porous product. This texture is a little more difficult to achieve when gluten-free flours, such as rice, maize and soy, are substituted for wheat flour.

This book is filled with delicious gluten-free recipes. Each recipe contains a nutritional analysis of the fat, protein, carbohydrate, fibre, cholesterol and energy content, as well as an estimated glycaemic index (GI) value for those who have diabetes.

The question of which ingredients can be eaten safely by people with coeliac disease continues to be debated worldwide. While it is acknowledged that some ingredients that contain very small amounts of gluten, such as wheat starch and oats, may be tolerated by some people with coeliac disease, they are not tolerated by all. The recipes in this book exclude many of the controversial ingredients. If your individual health condition requires specific dietary restrictions, the information in this book should not replace any advice given to you by your doctor or dietitian.

If you suspect you have coeliac disease or dermatitis herpetiformis, consult your doctor before making any dietary changes. Do not experiment with a gluten-free diet as you must be regularly eating foods that contain gluten in order to diagnose these conditions. Blood antibody tests can indicate whether or not you are likely to have coeliac disease, but only a biopsy of the small intestine can diagnose the condition.

WHAT IS COELIAC DISEASE?

Coeliac disease is a gastrointestinal disease, predominantly found in Caucasians. It can be diagnosed at any age, and tends to be hereditary, with a slight female predominance.

Coeliac disease is a condition where the lining (mucosa) of the small intestine becomes inflamed when gluten is ingested. The mucosa is covered with small finger-like projections called villi. The villi contain enzymes that help break down food. They also help transport nutrients from the small intestine into the bloodstream. When gluten is eaten by a person with coeliac disease, the villi become shortened and blunted or flat, resulting in the decreased absorption of all nutrients, protein, fat, carbohydrate, vitamins and minerals.

Symptoms of coeliac disease include weight loss, bloating, stomach cramps, diarrhoea, flatulence, nausea and vomiting. However, more subtle symptoms can also occur. Sometimes the only perceptible sign of the disease is iron deficiency. Headaches, tiredness, ataxia, mood disturbances, apparent food intolerances, enamel defects of permanent teeth, mouth ulcers, recurrent miscarriages, or general malaise may also suggest coeliac disease. This wide variety of signs and symptoms is often the reason for delayed diagnosis.

The damage to the villi is reversed, either totally or partially, by removing gluten from the diet. In untreated coeliac disease, the damaged villi and malabsorption of nutrients may result in persistent symptoms, anaemia and/or osteoporosis. There is also a greater chance of developing a cancer somewhere in the gastrointestinal tract, especially in the small intestine. The absorption of nutrients normalises between 6 and 12 months after starting a gluten-free diet. However, it takes about 5 years on a gluten-free diet before the cancer risk is decreased to the same level as that of the general population. People with coeliac disease are advised to follow a gluten-free diet for life in order to minimise all risks.

WHAT IS DERMATITIS HERPETIFORMIS?
Dermatitis herpetiformis (DH) is a gluten-sensitive, blistering skin disease. Found more often in males, these small, intensely itchy blisters are usually located around the elbows, knees and buttocks. DH can occur without underlying coeliac disease, but this is very uncommon. Many people with DH have few gastrointestinal symptoms, even though they also have coeliac disease. A skin biopsy is necessary to diagnose DH. Medication is usually given to control the rash in the short term. However, a gluten-free diet is recommended for lifelong control of the rash.

GLUTEN-FREE DIET
Corn (also known as maize), rice, soy, buckwheat, besan (chickpea), sorghum, potato, tapioca, sago and millet are just some of the gluten-free flours or grains available. Fresh milk, butter, cheese, fruit, vegetables, legumes, seeds, red meat, chicken and seafood are all gluten-free. Tea, coffee and wine can be consumed, but beer must be excluded.

Avoiding products made with wheat, triticale, rye, barley and oats may sound simple. However, many ingredients derived from these grains, such as the thickeners 1400-1450, hydrolysed vegetable protein, maltodextrin, malt and malt extract, contain small amounts of gluten. These ingredients can be found in products that otherwise seem to be gluten-free. In Australia, foods can only be labelled and sold as gluten-free if they do not contain oats, malt or detectable gluten. Currently, the lower limit for detecting gluten in foods is 20 parts per million, but the lower limit varies in different countries. In Australia, all commercially available foods must show on their label the grain from which any gluten-containing ingredients were derived, such as thickener 1442 (wheat). This helps people find out if there are any suspicious ingredients in products not labelled as gluten-free.

The Coeliac Society of Australia has produced an Ingredient List booklet to help identify gluten-free ingredients in foods. A dietitian can assist you with a gluten-free diet and advise you about which ingredients to avoid, as well as assess the nutritional adequacy of your overall diet.

GLUTEN-FREE GUIDELINES

If food is eaten from all 5 food groups, a gluten-free diet is able to provide a more than adequate nutritional intake.

1 | Be aware of gluten sources
Using gluten-free foods allows the villi to recover and good health to be restored.

2 | Be aware of fat sources
When the villi recover, more nutrients will be absorbed and some people gain a little weight. Maintaining low-fat cooking methods and low-fat food choices will help prevent this.

3 | Increase fibre intake
Maize cornflour and rice flour are the most frequently used flours in commercial gluten-free breads, pastas and snacks. These flours contain less fibre than wheat flour so special attention should be given to the fibre content of a gluten-free diet. Buckwheat, soy, brown rice and besan grains and flours are good sources of fibre to include in your home cooking. Legumes, nuts, seeds, fresh fruit and vegetables are other fibre sources. These foods also provide vitamins, minerals and other healthy compounds that can help reduce the risk of cancer.

4 | Be aware of calcium sources
Ensuring an adequate calcium intake is important to help prevent osteoporosis. Dairy foods are the best source of calcium. Choose 3 serves of dairy foods each day from milk, cheese or yoghurt. Other calcium sources include fortified soy milk, fish with edible bones, nuts and seeds.

5 | Be aware of iron and folate sources
Iron and folate deficiencies are often found at diagnosis and folate intakes are often low in a gluten-free diet. Many gluten-containing breads and breakfast cereals are fortified with iron and folate. However, very few commercial gluten-free products are fortified with extra nutrients. The best sources of iron are red and white meats, fish, eggs, legumes and nuts. The iron found in plant foods is not easily absorbed by the body. Good sources of folate include liver, cabbage, spinach, peanuts, peas and oranges.

6 | Choose alcohol wisely
Wine, spirits and liqueurs tend to be gluten-free. Beer should be avoided as it is made from malted barley and therefore contains small amounts of gluten. A recommended sensible intake of alcohol is 1-2 standard drinks per day.

Kim Faulkner-Hogg
(BSc, Grad Dip Nutr & Diet)

A GUIDE TO GLUTEN-FREE FOODS

SAFE FOODS*	FOODS TO AVOID*
Fresh fruit, vegetables, meat, poultry, seafood and eggs are gluten-free.	
Flours & grains Arrowroot | buckwheat | buckwheat flour | chickpea flour (besan) | cornmeal | lentil flour | maize cornflour | pea flour | polenta | potato flour | quinoa | rice (white and brown) | rice flour | ground rice | rice bran | glutinous rice | sago | tapioca | soy flour | wild rice | gluten-free baking powder	All varieties of wheat including bulgur, couscous, durum, kumat, spelt | wheat starch | wheaten cornflour | wheat flour | multigrain flour | wheatgerm | wheatmeal | wheat bran | semolina | triticale | rye | barley | oats | oatmeal | oat bran | malt | baking powder
Cereals Non-malted rice or corn breakfast cereals | baby rice cereal | gluten-free pasta | rice noodles | rice vermicelli	Wheat-based and mixed-grain breakfast cereals | muesli | rolled oats | baby cereals (except rice) | pasta | noodles | vermicelli
Breads, biscuits, cakes & pastries Gluten-free breads | taco shells | white corn tortillas | rice cakes and crackers (plain) | gluten-free biscuits, cakes and pastries	All breads, biscuits, cakes and pastries containing wheat, rye, barley or oats | sourdough commercial breads
Dairy & soy products Milk | calcium-fortified soy milk | baby formula | most yoghurts | cheese | plain ice cream | tofu	Malted milk | flavoured milk | custard powder | soy milk with malt/maltodextrin
Jams, spreads & condiments Jam | marmalade | honey | golden syrup | maple syrup | peanut butter | herbs | spices | curry powder | gluten-free tamari	Vegemite | Marmite | Promite | commercial relishes, chutneys and mustards | soy sauce
Beverages Water | rice milk | mineral water | soda water | tonic water | fruit juice | soft drinks | tea | coffee | wine | liqueurs | spirits	Coffee substitutes | drinking chocolate | malted drinks | oat milk | lemon barley | beers and ales

* Always check the ingredients of packaged and processed foods as ingredients may vary between manufacturers. Contact the Coeliac Society of Australia if you are unsure of any ingredient.

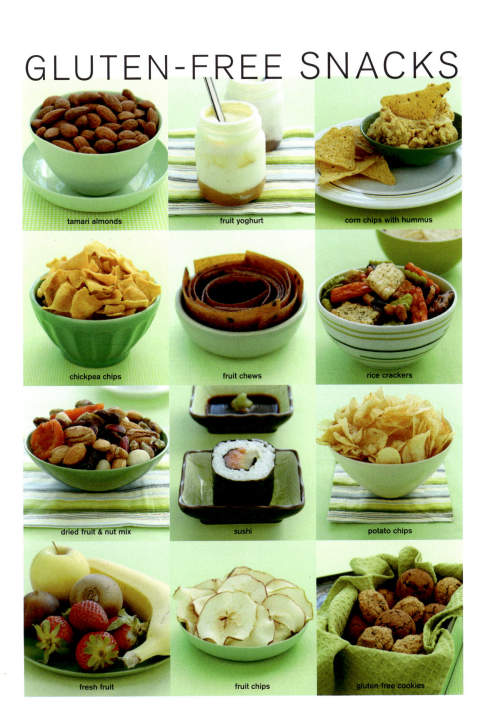

BREAKFAST

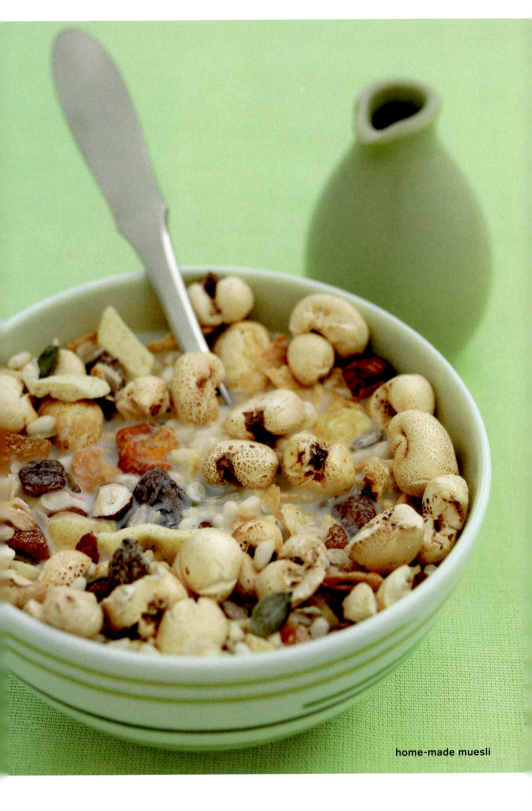

home-made muesli

HOME-MADE MUESLI

3 cups (30 g/1 oz) puffed corn cereal
2 cups (60 g/2 oz) puffed rice cereal
2 cups (50 g/1 2/3 oz) gluten-free rice flakes
1 cup (85 g/2 3/4 oz) psyllium husks
1 cup (120 g/4 oz) hazelnuts, roasted and roughly chopped
1 cup (140 g/4 1/2 oz) pepitas
1 cup (150 g/5 oz) sunflower seeds
2 cups (350 g/12 oz) mixed dried fruit

1 Put all of the ingredients into a large bowl and gently mix to combine.

2 Transfer the muesli to a large airtight container and seal until ready to use. Store in an airtight container for up to 2 months. Serve with soy milk and fresh fruit. Makes 11 cups

per cup | fat 20.6 g | saturated fat 2.2 g | protein 9.8 g | carbohydrate 33.7 g | fibre 12.2 g | cholesterol 0 mg | energy 1466 kJ (349 Cal) | gi 49 ▼ low

TEXAS-STYLE BEANS

300 g (10 oz) dried navy or haricot beans
2 teaspoons olive oil
1 medium onion, finely chopped
100 g (3 1/3 oz) trimmed bacon, finely chopped
800 g (1 lb 10 oz) can chopped tomatoes
1 tablespoon honey
1 teaspoon gluten-free Dijon mustard
1 tablespoon gluten-free Worcestershire sauce

1 Soak the beans overnight in cold water. Rinse the beans and put them into a large pan with 8 cups (2 litres/64 fl oz) water. Bring to the boil, then reduce the heat and simmer, covered, for 30 minutes. Drain the beans well.

2 Heat the oil in a heavy-based pan over medium heat. Add the onion and bacon and cook for 5 minutes or until the onion is soft.

3 Add the beans, tomatoes, honey, mustard and Worcestershire sauce. Cover and cook over medium heat for 45 minutes to 1 hour or until the sauce is thick. Serves 6

per serve | fat 4.4 g | saturated fat 0.9 g | protein 15.8 g | carbohydrate 29.3 g | fibre 11.1 g | cholesterol 10 mg | energy 980 kJ (233 Cal) | gi 33 ▼ low

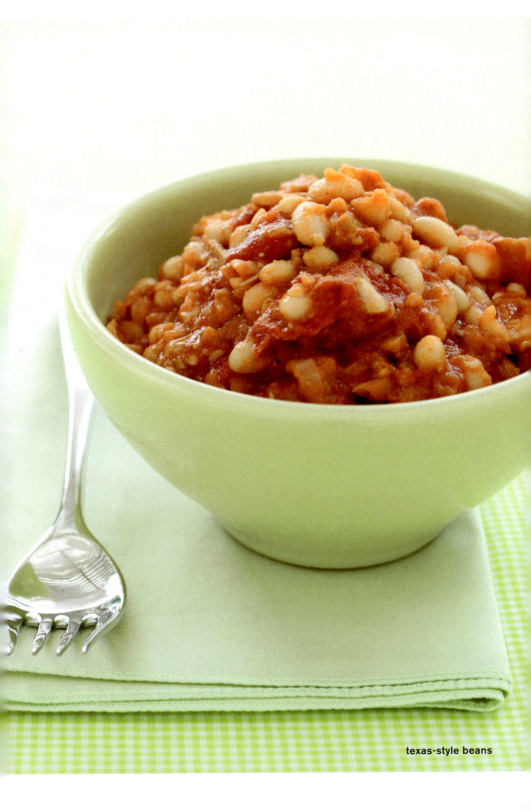

texas-style beans

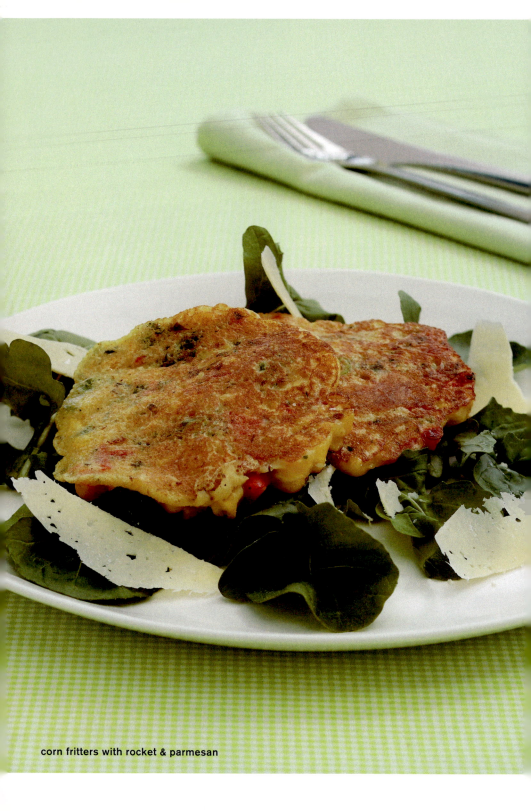
corn fritters with rocket & parmesan

CORN FRITTERS WITH ROCKET & PARMESAN

1 Sift the flour, baking powder and curry powder or turmeric into a bowl, stir in the sugar and make a well in the center.
2 Whisk together the eggs and milk. Gradually pour into the well and whisk to a smooth batter. Fold the corn kernels, capsicum, spring onions and herbs into the batter.
3 Heat the oil in a large non-stick fry pan over medium heat. Drop 2 tablespoons of the batter into the pan and cook for 3 minutes on each side or until golden and cooked through. Keep warm while you cook the remaining batter.
4 Serve the fritters with the rocket and parmesan, drizzled with balsamic vinegar. Serves 4

per serve | fat 13.7 g | saturated fat 4.1 g | protein 17.2 g | carbohydrate 46.5 g | fibre 7.6 g | cholesterol 107 mg | energy 1633 kJ (389 Cal) | gi 52 ▼ low

- 1 cup (120 g/4 oz) gluten-free all-purpose flour pre mix
- 1 teaspoon gluten-free baking powder
- ½ teaspoon gluten-free curry powder or turmeric (optional)
- 1 tablespoon sugar
- 2 eggs, lightly beaten
- ½ cup (125 ml/4 fl oz) skim or no-fat milk
- 2 cups (400 g/13 oz) fresh or frozen corn kernels
- 1 small red capsicum (bell pepper), chopped
- 4 spring onions (scallions), sliced
- 2 tablespoons chopped fresh herbs (parsley, chives, thyme)
- 1 tablespoon olive oil
- 100 g (3⅓ oz) rocket (arugula)
- 50 g (1⅔ oz) shaved parmesan cheese
- 2 tablespoons balsamic vinegar

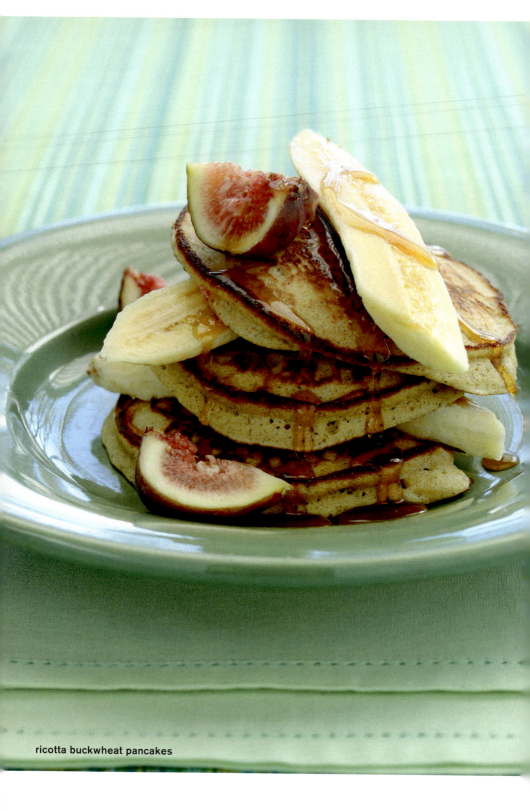

ricotta buckwheat pancakes

RICOTTA BUCKWHEAT PANCAKES

1 Sift the flour and baking powder into a bowl and stir in the sugar. Whisk together the ricotta, milk and egg yolks. Stir into the dry ingredients.
2 Whisk the egg whites in a clean, dry bowl until soft peaks form. Fold the egg whites into the batter.
3 Melt a little of the butter or margarine in a fry pan over medium heat. Pour 2 tablespoons of the batter into the pan and cook for 3 minutes or until bubbles appear on the surface. Turn the pancake over and cook the other side until golden. Keep warm while you cook the remaining batter.
4 Layer the sliced figs and bananas between the pancakes. Serve drizzled with maple syrup. Makes 8

per serve | fat 8.9 g | saturated fat 4.6 g | protein 11.6 g | carbohydrate 27.2 g | fibre 3.1 g | cholesterol 119 mg | energy 979 kJ (233 Cal) | gi 51 ▼ low

1 cup (120 g/4 oz) buckwheat flour
1 teaspoon gluten-free baking powder
2 tablespoons caster sugar
340 g (11¼ oz) low-fat ricotta cheese
¾ cup (185 ml/6 fl oz) skim or no-fat milk
4 eggs, separated
20 g (¾ oz) butter or canola margarine
4 fresh figs, quartered
4 medium bananas, sliced
maple syrup, to serve

HAM, EGG & TOMATO QUESADILLAS

1 Heat a little of the butter or margarine in a non-stick fry pan. Cook the eggs one at a time until done to your liking.
2 Lay 4 of the tortillas on a flat surface. Divide the ham, eggs, tomatoes and cheese among the tortillas. Top with the remaining tortillas.
3 Melt a little of the remaining butter or margarine in a non-stick fry pan, add a tortilla stack and weigh it down with a plate. Cook over medium heat for 2 minutes or until the bottom tortilla is crisp and golden.
4 Slide the tortilla out of the pan and onto a plate. Return to the pan and cook the other side until crisp and golden. Keep warm while you cook the remaining tortillas. Cut into wedges to serve. Serves 4

per serve | fat 13.3 g | saturated fat 5.2 g | protein 15.3 g | carbohydrate 9.6 g | fibre 2 g | cholesterol 215 mg | energy 933 kJ (222 Cal) | gi 47 ▼ low

30 g (1 oz) butter or reduced-fat margarine
4 eggs
8 medium gluten-free white corn tortillas
100 g (3⅓ oz) sliced 97% fat-free ham
2 medium tomatoes, sliced
3 tablespoons grated reduced-fat cheddar cheese

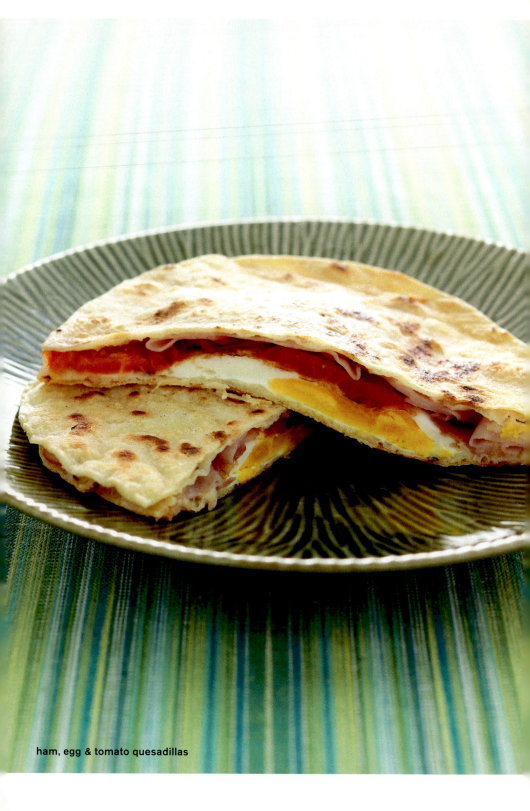
ham, egg & tomato quesadillas

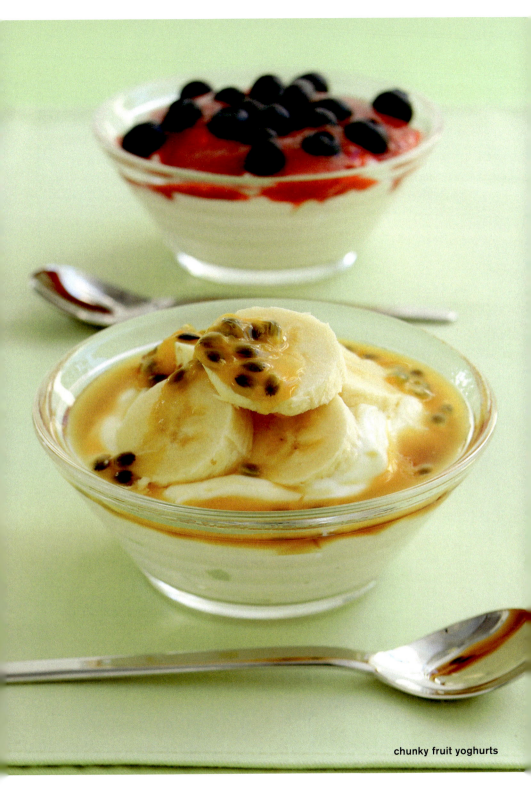

chunky fruit yoghurts

CHUNKY FRUIT YOGHURTS

BANANA & PASSIONFRUIT
400 g (13 oz) reduced-fat Greek-style plain yoghurt
2 tablespoons maple syrup*
2 medium bananas, sliced
¼ cup (60 ml/2 fl oz) passionfruit pulp

BERRY DELIGHT
200 g (6½ oz) strawberries
1 tablespoon yellow box honey
400 g (13 oz) reduced-fat Greek-style plain yoghurt
300 g (10 oz) mixed fresh berries

1 To make banana & passionfruit yoghurt, divide the yoghurt among 4 bowls and top with the maple syrup, bananas and passionfruit. Serves 4

2 To make berry delight yoghurt, put the strawberries and honey into a blender or food processor and process until smooth. Divide the yoghurt among 4 bowls and top with the strawberry mixture and mixed berries. Serves 4

per serve (banana & passionfruit) | fat 1.8 g | saturated fat 1.1 g | protein 6.3 g | carbohydrate 27.5 g | fibre 3.3 g | cholesterol 10 mg | energy 676 kJ (161 Cal) | gi 42 ▼ low

per serve (berry delight) | fat 1.8 g | saturated fat 1.1 g | protein 7.1 g | carbohydrate 17.2 g | fibre 2.8 g | cholesterol 10 mg | energy 518 kJ (123 Cal) | gi 27 ▼ low

* If you have diabetes, you could either reduce the maple syrup or replace it with a little yellow box honey in order to lower the blood sugar response to this dish.

POLENTA PORRIDGE

4 cups (1 litre/32 fl oz) skim or no-fat milk
1 cup (150 g/5 oz) fine polenta (cornmeal)
¼ cup (60 g/2 oz) caster sugar
1 teaspoon orange-flower water
200 g (6½ oz) reduced-fat Greek-style plain yoghurt
200 g (6½ oz) strawberries, halved
100 g (3⅓ oz) blueberries
2 tablespoons maple syrup

1 Put the milk into a pan and stir over medium heat until it is almost boiling. Gradually whisk in the polenta and stir for 5 minutes or until the porridge starts to thicken. Remove from the heat.

2 Stir the sugar and orange-flower water into the porridge. Cover and set aside for 5 minutes.

3 Spoon the porridge into 6 serving bowls, top with the yoghurt and berries and drizzle with the maple syrup. Serves 6

per serve | fat 1.2 g | saturated fat 0.6 g | protein 10.3 g | carbohydrate 43.5 g | fibre 1.7 g | cholesterol 9 mg | energy 957 kJ (228 Cal) | gi 52 ▼ low

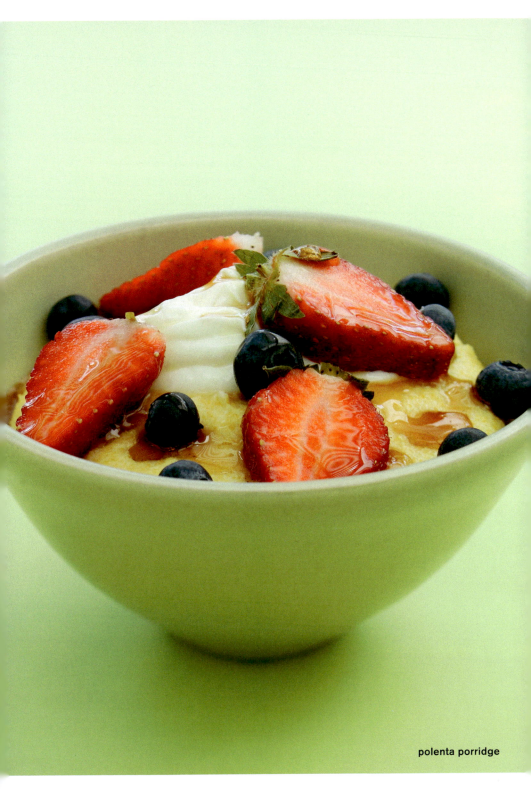

polenta porridge

LUNCH & DINNER

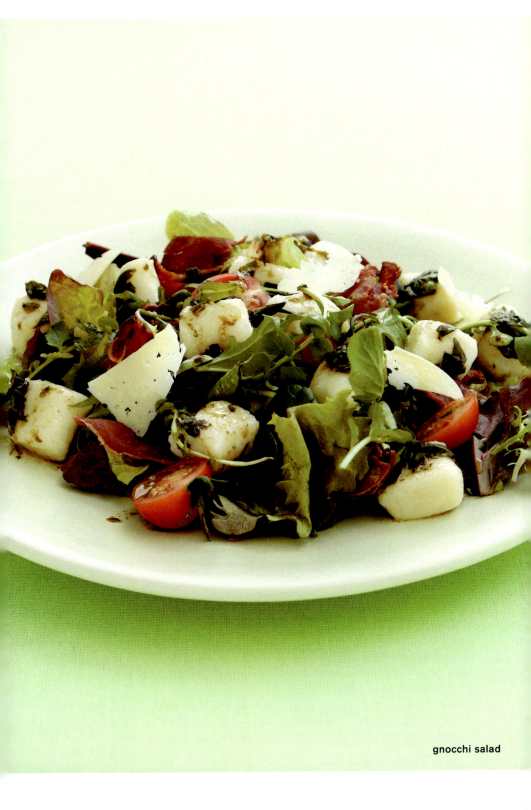

gnocchi salad

GNOCCHI SALAD

750 g (1½ lb) floury potatoes, peeled and chopped
½ cup (50 g/1⅔ oz) finely grated parmesan cheese
1 cup (120 g/4 oz) gluten-free all-purpose flour pre mix
⅓ cup (20 g/¾ oz) baby rice cereal
250 g (8 oz) cherry tomatoes, halved
100 g (3⅓ oz) mixed salad leaves
50 g (1⅔ oz) prosciutto, grilled
2 tablespoons extra virgin olive oil
2 tablespoons balsamic vinegar
cracked black pepper
20 g (¾ oz) shaved parmesan cheese

1 Cook the potatoes in a large pan of boiling water until soft. Drain well, return to the pan and cook over medium heat until there is no moisture left in the pan.
2 Mash the potatoes. Add the grated parmesan, flour and rice cereal and mix to a soft dough. Gather into a ball and cut into quarters. Shape each quarter into a cylinder. Cut each cylinder into 3 cm (1¼ in) pieces.
3 Cook the gnocchi in batches in a large pan of rapidly boiling water until they float to the surface. Cook for 1 minute, then remove with a slotted spoon and keep warm while you cook the remaining gnocchi.
4 Toss the gnocchi with the tomatoes, salad leaves and prosciutto. Drizzle with the olive oil and vinegar, and sprinkle with the pepper and parmesan. Serves 6

per serve | fat 10.3 g | saturated fat 3.1 g | protein 11.1 g | carbohydrate 33.8 g | fibre 4.2 g | cholesterol 14 mg | energy 1184 kJ (282 Cal) | gi 65 ◆ med

SPICY TUNA TACOS

500 g (1 lb) tuna, thickly sliced
2 teaspoons Tabasco sauce
½ teaspoon cracked black pepper
1 tablespoon lime juice
3 small tomatoes, chopped
1 red (Spanish) onion, chopped
1 tablespoon capers, chopped
1 medium avocado, chopped
1 tablespoon chopped fresh coriander (cilantro)
8 gluten-free corn taco shells
2 teaspoons olive oil
2 cups (115 g/3⅔ oz) shredded lettuce
200 g (6½ oz) reduced-fat Greek-style plain yoghurt

1 Preheat oven to 180°C (350°F/Gas 4).
2 Put the tuna, Tabasco, pepper and lime juice into a bowl and mix to combine. Marinate for 15 minutes.
3 Put the tomatoes, onion, capers, avocado and coriander into a bowl and mix to combine.
4 Arrange the taco shells on a baking tray and bake for 10 minutes or until heated through.
5 Meanwhile, heat the oil in a large non-stick fry pan over high heat. Cook the tuna for 5 minutes each side or until browned and tender.
6 Divide the tuna among the taco shells. Top with the lettuce and the tomato mixture and finish with a dollop of yoghurt. Serves 4

per serve | fat 30 g | saturated fat 7.6 g | protein 38.8 g | carbohydrate 22.3 g | fibre 5.4 g | cholesterol 50 mg | energy 2167 kJ (516 Cal) | gi 50 ▼ low

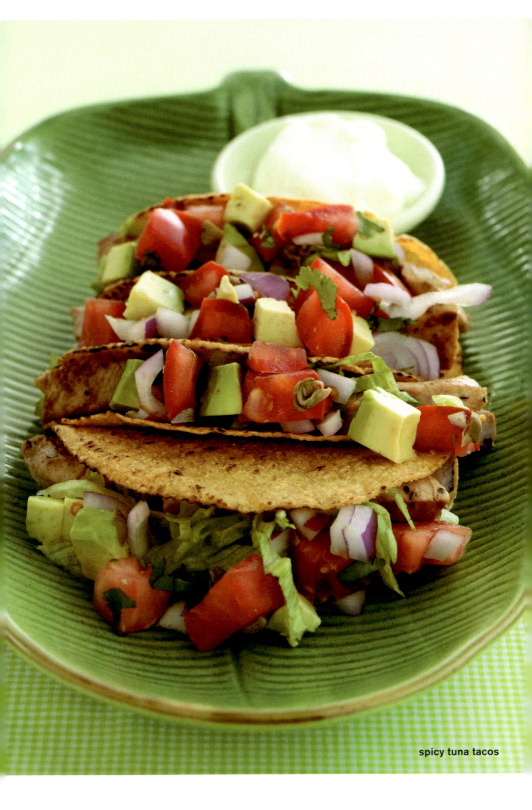
spicy tuna tacos

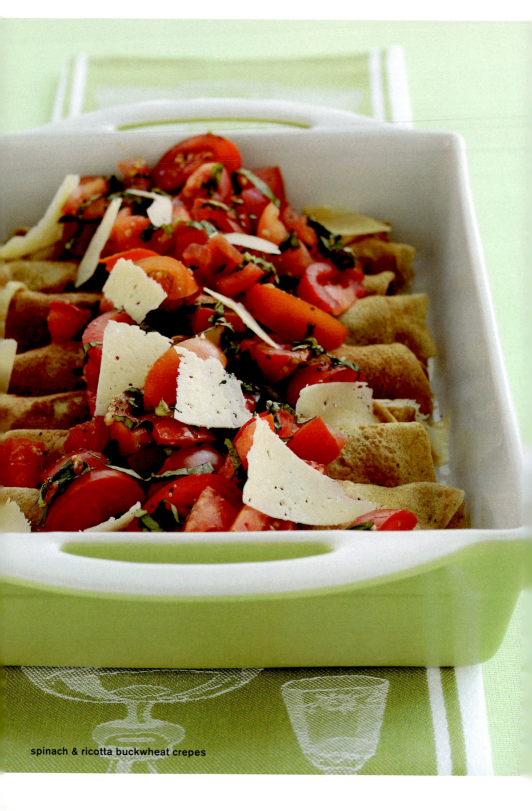
spinach & ricotta buckwheat crepes

SPINACH & RICOTTA BUCKWHEAT CREPES

1 Preheat oven to 180°C (350°F/Gas 4).
2 Sift the flours into a bowl and make a well in the center. Whisk together the milk, water, eggs and oil and pour into the well.
3 Lightly spray a small non-stick fry pan with canola oil spray. Pour 2 tablespoons of the batter into the pan and tilt to cover the base with the batter. Cook over medium heat for 2 minutes or until the crepe is golden on the underside. Turn the crepe over and cook the other side until golden. Repeat with the remaining batter.
4 Wash the spinach and put into a pan. Cover and cook over medium heat for 5 minutes or until wilted. Leave to cool slightly, then squeeze out any excess moisture. Roughly chop the spinach.
5 Put the spinach, ricotta and nutmeg into a bowl and mix to combine. Season with salt and pepper. Place 2 tablespoons of the mixture along the center of each crepe and roll up to enclose the filling. Arrange the crepes in an ovenproof dish and bake for 20 minutes or until heated through.
6 Put the tomatoes, garlic and basil into a bowl, mix to combine and season generously with salt and pepper. Spoon over the center of the crepes and top with the parmesan shavings. Serve with a mixed green salad. Serves 4

½ cup (60 g/2 oz) buckwheat flour
½ cup (60 g/2 oz) gluten-free all-purpose flour pre mix
1 cup (250 ml/8 fl oz) skim or no-fat milk
⅔ cup (170 ml/5½ fl oz) water
3 eggs, lightly beaten
2 tablespoons canola oil
canola oil spray
750 g (1½ lb) English spinach, trimmed
200 g (6½ oz) reduced-fat ricotta cheese
½ teaspoon ground nutmeg
salt and pepper
400 g (13 oz) tomatoes, cut into wedges
2 cloves garlic, crushed
2 tablespoons finely shredded fresh basil
50 g (1⅔ oz) shaved parmesan cheese

per serve | fat 23.5 g | saturated fat 7.4 g | protein 25.9 g | carbohydrate 29 g | fibre 9.1 g | cholesterol 176 mg | energy 1787 kJ (425 Cal) | gi 46 ▼ low

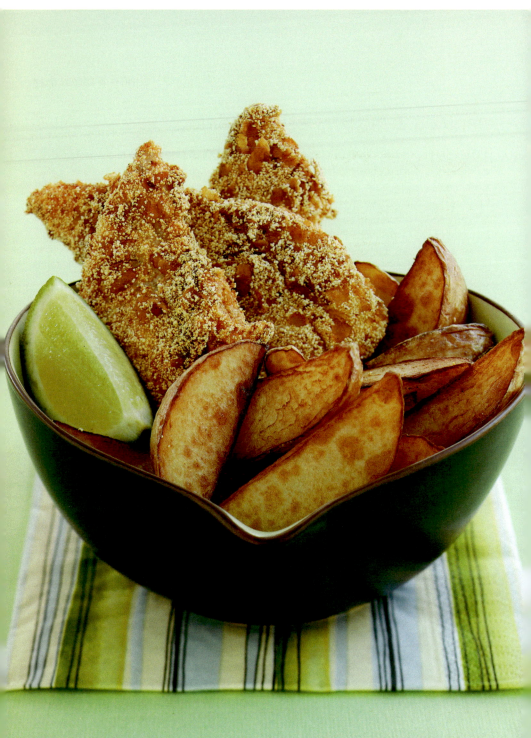
crunchy polenta fish & chips

CRUNCHY POLENTA FISH & CHIPS

1 Combine the polenta, rice flakes, paprika and lemon zest in a shallow bowl.
2 Dip the fish fillets into the egg whites, then coat in the polenta mixture, shaking off any excess.
3 Heat the oil in a wok or heavy-based pan over medium heat for 5 minutes or until the oil starts to move. Stand a wooden chopstick in the oil. If the oil bubbles around the chopstick, it is ready.
4 Cook the fish in batches in the oil until crisp and golden. Drain on absorbent paper and keep warm.
5 Cook the potatoes in batches in the oil until crisp and golden. Drain on absorbent paper. Serve the fish and chips with lime wedges. Serves 4

per serve | fat 8.2 g | saturated fat 1.9 g | protein 42.7 g | carbohydrate 47.5 g | fibre 4.2 g | cholesterol 101 mg | energy 1875 kJ (446 Cal) | gi 68 ◆ med

1 cup (150 g/5 oz) fine polenta (cornmeal)
1 cup (25 g/1 oz) gluten-free rice flakes
1 teaspoon mild paprika
1 teaspoon lemon zest
4 boneless white fish fillets
3 egg whites, lightly beaten
peanut oil for deep frying
500 g (1 lb) potatoes, unpeeled and cut into wedges
lime wedges

SPINACH, TOMATO & FETTA PASTA FRITTATAS

1 Preheat oven to 180°C (350°F/Gas 4). Lightly grease a 6 x 1 cup (250 ml/8 fl oz) capacity non-stick muffin pan.
2 Cook the pasta in a large pan of rapidly boiling water for 5 minutes or until just tender, then drain well.
3 Wash the spinach and put into a pan. Cover and cook over medium heat for 5 minutes or until wilted. Cool, then squeeze out any moisture and roughly chop.
4 Whisk together the eggs, milk, parmesan and basil.
5 Divide the pasta among the muffin holes and arrange the spinach, fetta and tomatoes on top. Pour in the egg mixture and swirl gently with a skewer so the egg reaches the bottom. Bake for 20 minutes or until set. Serve hot or cold with salad. Serves 6

per serve | fat 11 g | saturated fat 4.4 g | protein 22.2 g | carbohydrate 24.8 g | fibre 3.5 g | cholesterol 264 mg | energy 1231 kJ (293 Cal) | gi 46 ▼ low

200 g (6½ oz) gluten-free rice and legume pasta spirals
250 g (8 oz) English spinach, trimmed
8 eggs, lightly beaten
½ cup (125 ml/4 fl oz) reduced-fat evaporated milk
2 tablespoons grated parmesan cheese
2 tablespoons chopped fresh basil
100 g (3⅓ oz) reduced-fat fetta cheese, broken into large pieces
100 g (3⅓ oz) semi-dried tomatoes, roughly chopped

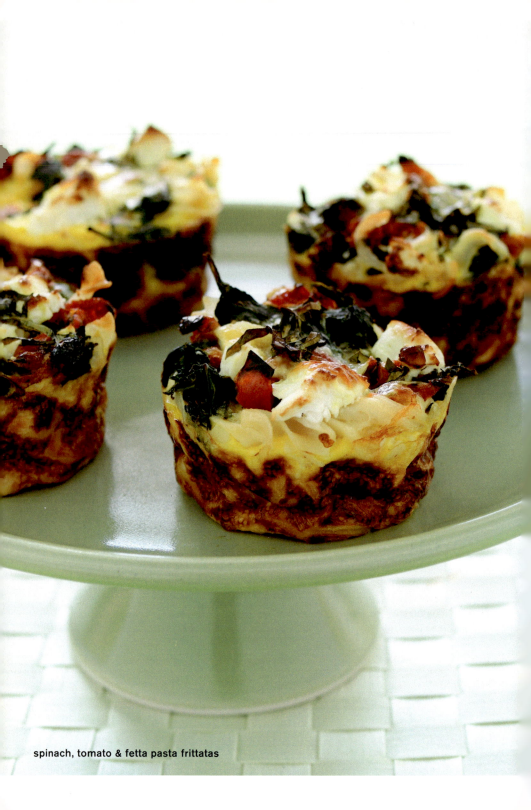
spinach, tomato & fetta pasta frittatas

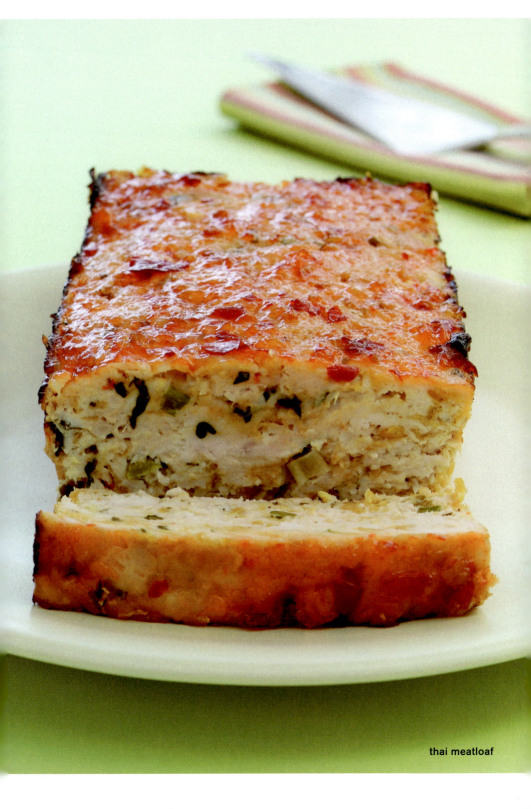

thai meatloaf

THAI MEATLOAF

1 kg (2 lb) chicken mince
1 cup (30 g/1 oz) gluten-free cornflakes
4 spring onions (scallions), sliced
1 tablespoon finely grated fresh ginger
2 tablespoons chopped fresh coriander (cilantro)
1 egg, lightly beaten
2 tablespoons fish sauce
1/3 cup (80 ml/2 2/3 fl oz) gluten-free sweet chilli sauce

1 Preheat oven to 180°C (350°F/Gas 4).
2 Put the chicken, cornflakes, spring onions, ginger, coriander, egg, fish sauce and 2 tablespoons of the sweet chilli sauce into a bowl and mix to combine.
3 Spoon the mixture into a 10 cm x 23 cm (4 in x 9 in) non-stick loaf tin and press down firmly.
4 Spread the remaining sweet chilli sauce over the loaf and bake for 30-40 minutes or until tender. Drain off any excess liquid. Serve the meatloaf hot or cold with salad or vegetables or on thick slices of mixed grain bread with Asian salad leaves. Serves 6
per serve | fat 14.6 g | saturated fat 4.3 g | protein 34.3 g | carbohydrate 9.7 g | fibre 0.5 g | cholesterol 181 mg | energy 1284 kJ (306 Cal) | gi 47 ▼ low

PRAWN RICE PAPER ROLLS

100 g (3 1/3 oz) dried rice vermicelli
20 rice paper rounds, 16 cm (6 1/2 in) diameter
20 cooked medium king prawns, peeled, deveined and halved
40 fresh mint leaves
2 cups (115 g/3 2/3 oz) finely shredded lettuce
1 large red chilli, seeded and finely chopped
2 tablespoons fish sauce
2 tablespoons lime juice
1 tablespoon brown sugar

1 Put the vermicelli into a bowl, cover with boiling water and allow to stand for 10 minutes or until the noodles are soft. Drain well. Cut into shorter pieces.
2 Soak a rice paper round in lukewarm water until soft. Place on a clean work surface.
3 Place a heaped tablespoon of the noodles along one edge of the rice paper round and top with 2 prawn halves, 2 mint leaves and some lettuce.
4 Fold in the sides and roll up to enclose the filling. Place on a plate and cover with damp absorbent paper while you prepare the remaining rolls.
5 Put the chilli, fish sauce, lime juice and sugar in a bowl and stir until the sugar has dissolved. Serve the rolls with the dipping sauce. Makes 20
per roll | fat 0.3 g | saturated fat 0.03 g | protein 4.5 g | carbohydrate 6.3 g | fibre 0.4 g | cholesterol 30 mg | energy 194 kJ (46 Cal) | gi 55 ▼ low
* The rolls will keep in an airtight container, separated with baking paper, for up to 2 days.

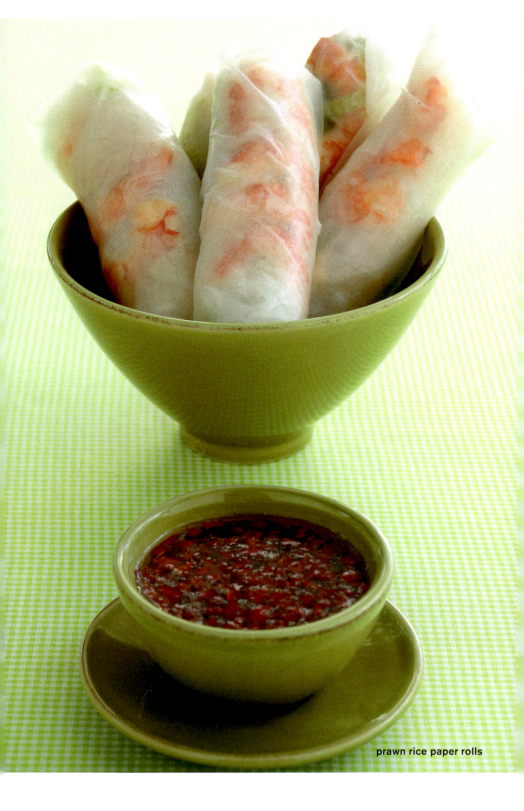
prawn rice paper rolls

CARAMELISED ONION & FETTA QUICHE

½ cup (60 g/2 oz) gluten-free all-purpose flour pre mix
1½ cups (90 g/3 oz) baby rice cereal
125 g (4 oz) butter or reduced-fat margarine
1 egg white
1-2 tablespoons iced water
1 tablespoon oil
500 g (1 lb) onions, thinly sliced
1 tablespoon balsamic vinegar
3 eggs, lightly beaten
¾ cup (185 ml/6 fl oz) milk
¼ cup (30 g/1 oz) grated cheddar cheese
2 teaspoons fresh thyme leaves
150 g (5 oz) reduced-fat fetta cheese, broken into bite-size pieces

1 Put the flour and rice cereal into a bowl and rub in the butter or margarine until the mixture resembles fine breadcrumbs. Add the egg white and iced water and stir into the dry ingredients using a flat-bladed knife. Mix until the pastry just comes together.

2 Gather the pastry into a ball and flatten slightly. Roll out between 2 large sheets of baking paper to cover the base and side of a 20 cm (8 in) ovenproof ceramic or glass pie dish. Fit the pastry into the tin, trimming off any excess pastry with a sharp knife. Chill for 20 minutes.

3 Preheat oven to 200°C (400°F/Gas 6).

4 Heat the oil in a large non-stick fry pan over low-medium heat, add the onions and balsamic vinegar and cook for 20 minutes or until the onions are caramelised. Set aside to cool slightly.

5 Cover the chilled pastry with baking paper and fill with uncooked rice or baking beads. Bake for 15 minutes, then remove the rice or beads and paper and cook for a further 5 minutes or until golden.

6 Spoon the onions into the pastry base. Whisk together the eggs, milk, cheese and thyme and pour over the onions. Sprinkle the fetta over the top. Bake for 40 minutes or until set. Serves 6

per serve I fat 23.3 g I saturated fat 12 g I protein 15.8 g I carbohydrate 23.3 g I fibre 2.2 g I cholesterol 145 mg I energy 1705 kJ (406 Cal) I gi 61 ♦ med

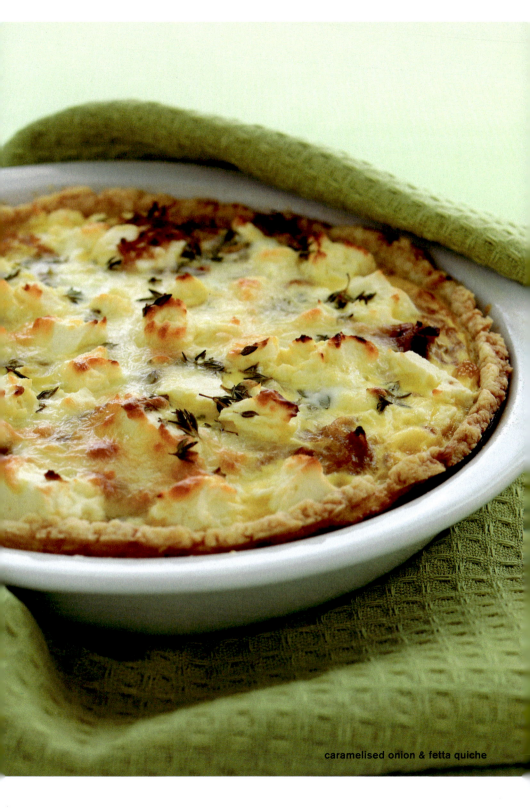
caramelised onion & fetta quiche

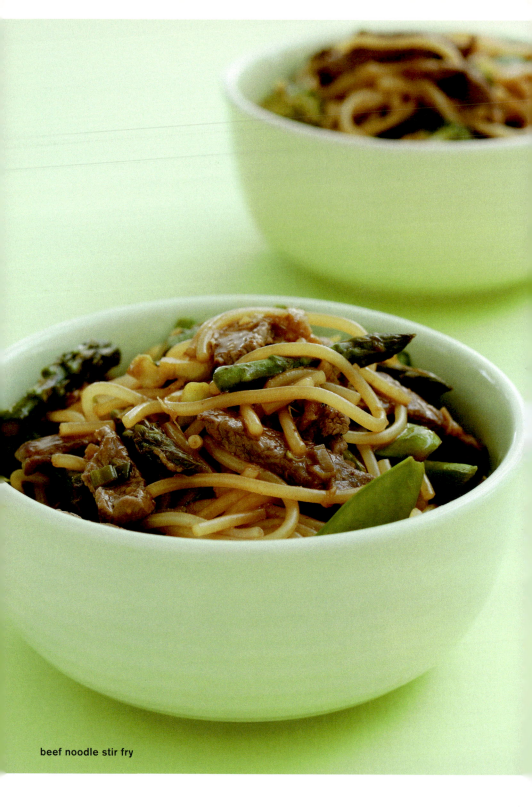
beef noodle stir fry

BEEF NOODLE STIR FRY

1 Heat the oil in a wok over high heat, add the steak and stir fry until browned.
2 Add the garlic, grated ginger, spring onions and 2 tablespoons of the water and stir fry for 3 minutes. Add the vegetables and remaining water and stir fry for 3 minutes or until the vegetables are bright green.
3 Add the noodles and stir fry for 2 minutes or until they begin to soften.
4 Add the tamari, mirin, sake and sugar to the wok and stir until the sauce boils and thickens. Serves 4
per serve | fat 9.2 g | saturated fat 2.7 g | protein 37.2 g | carbohydrate 30.8 g | fibre 7.2 g | cholesterol 80 mg | energy 1573 kJ (375 Cal) | gi 36 ▼ low

2 teaspoons canola oil
500 g (1 lb) lean rump steak, sliced
2 cloves garlic, chopped
1 tablespoon grated fresh ginger
4 spring onions (scallions), sliced
100 ml (3⅓ fl oz) water
200 g (6½ oz) snowpeas
300 g (10 oz) asparagus, chopped
200 g (6½ oz) broccoli, cut into florets
1 medium red capsicum (bell pepper), sliced
100 g (3⅓ oz) fresh baby corn
300 g (10 oz) fresh gluten-free rice noodles, separated
¼ cup (60 ml/2 fl oz) gluten-free tamari
1 tablespoon mirin
1 tablespoon sake
1 tablespoon sugar

SWEET CHILLI CHICKEN WRAPS

1 Lay the tortillas on a work surface.
2 Remove and discard the skin from the chicken and slice the meat.
3 Divide the chicken, spinach, cheese, sweet chilli sauce and yoghurt among the tortillas and roll up.
4 Heat a sandwich press and lightly spray it with olive oil spray. Cook the wraps for 3-5 minutes or until crisp and golden. Serves 4
per serve | fat 7.3 g | saturated fat 2.4 g | protein 20.8 g | carbohydrate 10.4 g | fibre 1.6 g | cholesterol 61 mg | energy 815 kJ (194 Cal) | gi 44 ▼ low

4 medium gluten-free white corn tortillas
½ barbecue chicken
30 g (1 oz) baby English spinach
2 tablespoons grated reduced-fat cheddar cheese
2 tablespoons gluten-free sweet chilli sauce
2 tablespoons plain yoghurt
olive oil spray

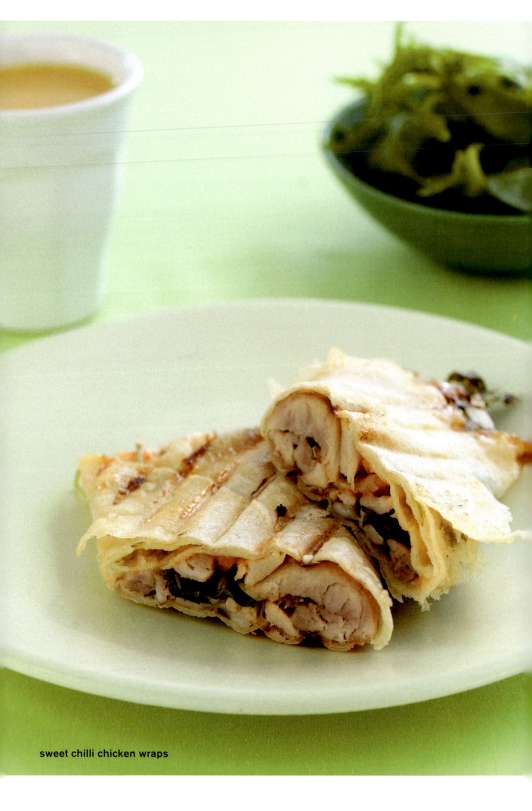

sweet chilli chicken wraps

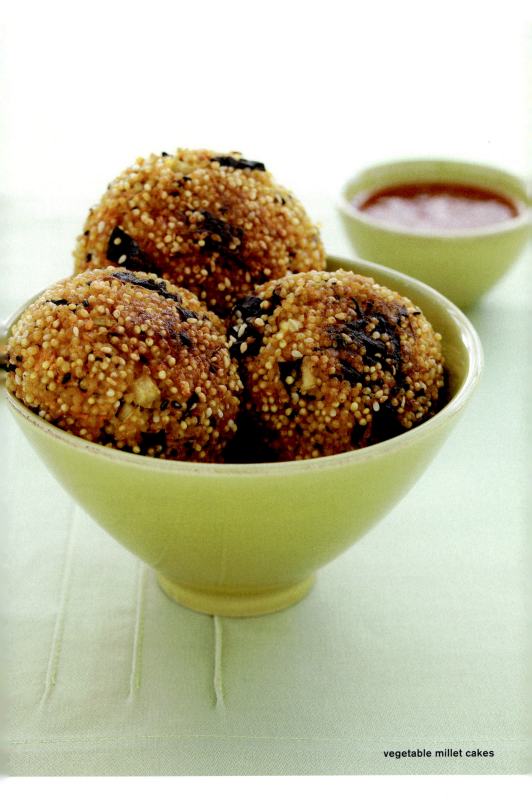
vegetable millet cakes

VEGETABLE MILLET CAKES

1 cup (210 g/6¾ oz) millet
2½ cups (625 ml/20 fl oz) gluten-free vegetable stock made from a stock cube
1 carrot, finely grated
1 celery stick, finely chopped
2 tablespoons sesame seeds
2 sheets (10 g/⅓ oz) nori seaweed, cut into thin strips
100 ml (3⅓ fl oz) gluten-free tamari
⅓ cup (20 g/¾ oz) baby rice cereal
2 tablespoons olive oil
1 tablespoon lemon juice

1 Put the millet and stock into a pan and bring to the boil over high heat. Reduce the heat and simmer for 20 minutes or until nearly all the liquid has been absorbed. Remove from the heat, cover and set aside for 10 minutes.
2 Stir the carrot, celery, sesame seeds, nori and 2 tablespoons of the tamari into the millet. Cover and set aside for 5 minutes. Stir in the rice cereal.
3 Preheat oven to 180°C (350°F/Gas 4). Line a baking tray with baking paper.
4 Shape the millet mixture into 8 balls.
5 Heat the oil in a large non-stick fry pan over medium heat. Cook a few millet cakes at a time for 3 minutes each side or until crisp and golden. Transfer to the prepared baking tray and bake for 15 minutes or until heated through.
6 Combine the lemon juice and remaining tamari. Serve the millet cakes with the dipping sauce.
Makes 8
per cake | fat 7.6 g | saturated fat 1.2 g | protein 5.5 g | carbohydrate 20.2 g | fibre 3.2 g | cholesterol 0 mg | energy 762 kJ (181 Cal) | gi 65 ◆ med

INDIAN CHICKEN DRUMSTICKS

8 (1.25 kg/2½ lb) chicken drumsticks
1 tablespoon madras curry paste
1 tablespoon honey
2 teaspoons lemon juice
200 g (6½ oz) reduced-fat Greek-style plain yoghurt

1 Make 2 deep incisions on either side of each drumstick and put into a non-metallic ovenproof dish.
2 Combine the curry paste, honey, lemon juice and yoghurt. Spoon over the drumsticks and gently toss to coat. Cover and marinate in the fridge for 4 hours.
3 Preheat oven to 220°C (425°F/Gas 7).
4 Bake the drumsticks for 40 minutes or until tender. Serve with saffron rice and vegetables. Makes 8
per drumstick | fat 18.4 g | saturated fat 5.5 g | protein 28.6 g | carbohydrate 5.1 g | fibre 0.3 g | cholesterol 164 mg | energy 1257 kJ (299 Cal) | gi 35 ▼ low

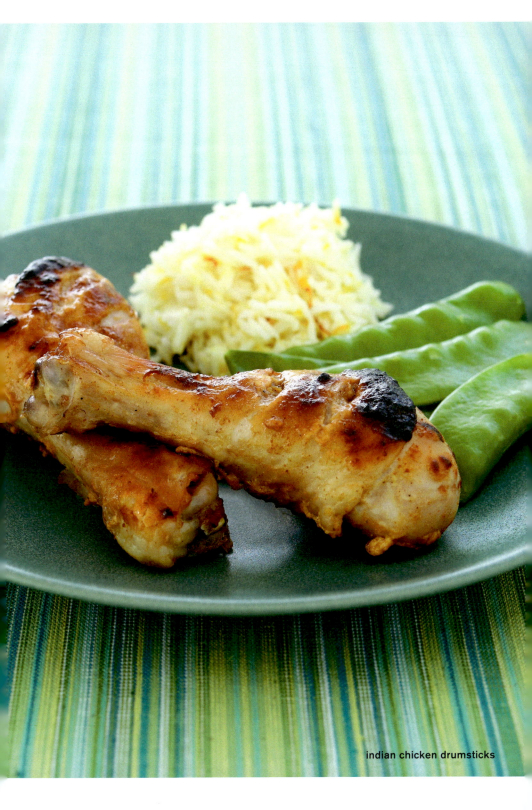

indian chicken drumsticks

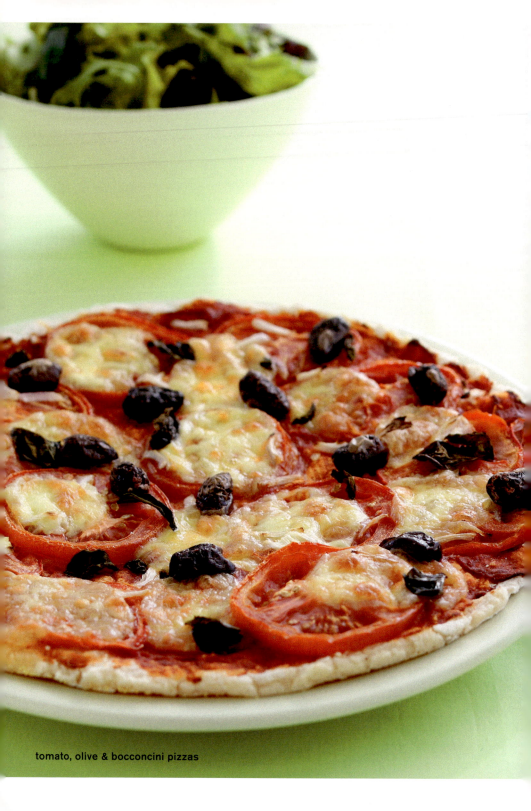
tomato, olive & bocconcini pizzas

TOMATO, OLIVE & BOCCONCINI PIZZAS

1 Sprinkle a pizza tray with polenta.
2 Combine the flour, salt, sugar and yeast in a bowl. Make a well in the center, add the combined water and oil and mix until the dough comes together.
3 Turn the dough out on a lightly floured surface and knead for 5 minutes or until smooth. Transfer to a large lightly oiled bowl and turn the dough to coat in the oil. Cover with plastic wrap and set aside in a warm place to rise for 1 hour or until the dough has doubled in size.
4 Preheat oven to 230°C (450°F/Gas 8).
5 Punch down the dough in the center and roll out on a lightly floured surface or between 2 sheets of baking paper until almost large enough to fit the pizza tray. Use your fingers to press the dough to fit the tray, pressing it together if it breaks.
6 Spread the pizza base with tomato paste and top with the tomato, onion, bocconcini, olives and basil. Bake for 15 minutes or until the dough is crisp and golden. Serves 2

per serve | fat 16 g | saturated fat 5.7 g | protein 19.8 g | carbohydrate 78.1 g | fibre 10.3 g | cholesterol 18 mg | **energy 2338 kJ (557 Cal)** | gi 53 ▼ low

polenta (cornmeal), to sprinkle
1 １/２ cups (180 g/6 oz) gluten-free all-purpose flour pre mix
１/２ teaspoon salt
1 teaspoon sugar
1 teaspoon dried yeast
150 ml (5 fl oz) lukewarm water
2 teaspoons olive oil
2 tablespoons tomato paste
2 medium ripe tomatoes, sliced
１/２ red (Spanish) onion, thinly sliced
100 g (3 １/３ oz) bocconcini (small, fresh mozzarella cheese), sliced
50 g (1 ２/３ oz) kalamata olives
30 g (1 oz) fresh basil leaves

POLENTA BOLOGNESE BAKE

4 cups (1 litre/32 fl oz) water
1 cup (150 g/5 oz) fine polenta (cornmeal)
¼ cup (25 g/1 oz) finely grated parmesan cheese
20 g (¾ oz) butter, chopped
2 teaspoons chopped fresh rosemary
2 teaspoons olive oil
1 medium onion, chopped
2 cloves garlic, crushed
500 g (1 lb) lean beef mince
400 g (13 oz) can chopped tomatoes
1 cup (250 ml/8 fl oz) red wine
1 tablespoon tomato paste
1 tablespoon brown sugar
200 g (6½ oz) reduced-fat ricotta cheese
150 ml (5 fl oz) reduced-fat evaporated milk
salt and pepper
½ cup (60 g/2 oz) grated reduced-fat cheddar cheese

1 Put the water into a pan and bring to the boil. Reduce the heat and gradually whisk in the polenta. Cook, whisking constantly for 10 minutes, then cook for a further 25 minutes, stirring occasionally with a wooden spoon until the polenta is thick enough for a spoon to stand upright in the center.
2 Stir the parmesan, butter and rosemary into the polenta. Spoon into a 10 cup (2.5 litre/80 fl oz) capacity ovenproof dish, cover and set aside.
3 Preheat oven to 180°C (350°F/Gas 4).
4 Heat the oil in a large non-stick fry pan over medium heat, add the onion and garlic and cook for 5 minutes or until the onion is golden.
5 Add the beef and cook, stirring, until browned. Stir in the tomatoes, wine, tomato paste and brown sugar. Bring to the boil and cook for 5 minutes to evaporate the alcohol. Reduce the heat and simmer for 15-20 minutes or until the sauce has thickened. Spoon the bolognese sauce over the polenta.
6 Combine the ricotta and evaporated milk and season with salt and pepper. Drop spoonfuls of the mixture on top of the bolognese sauce. Sprinkle with the grated cheese and bake for 40 minutes or until the cheese is golden. Serves 8

per serve | fat 12.9 g | saturated fat 6.5 g | protein 22.2 g | carbohydrate 18.2 g | fibre 1.6 g | cholesterol 58 mg | energy 1245 kJ (296 Cal) | gi 52 ▼ low

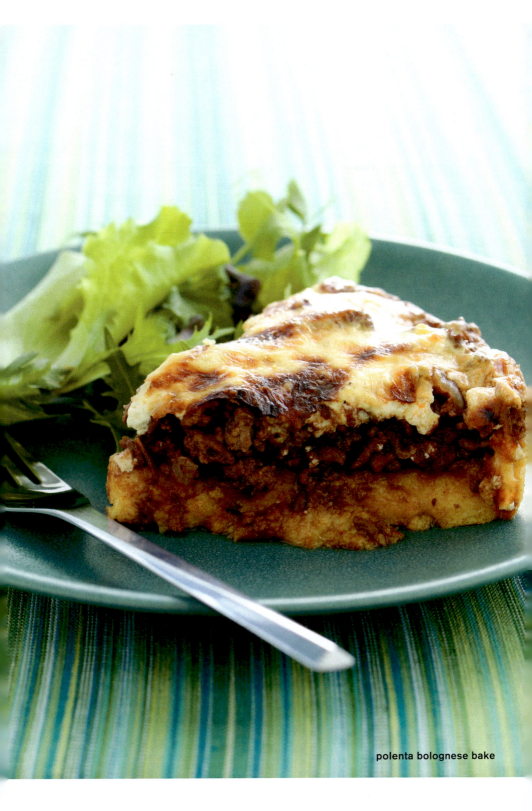

polenta bolognese bake

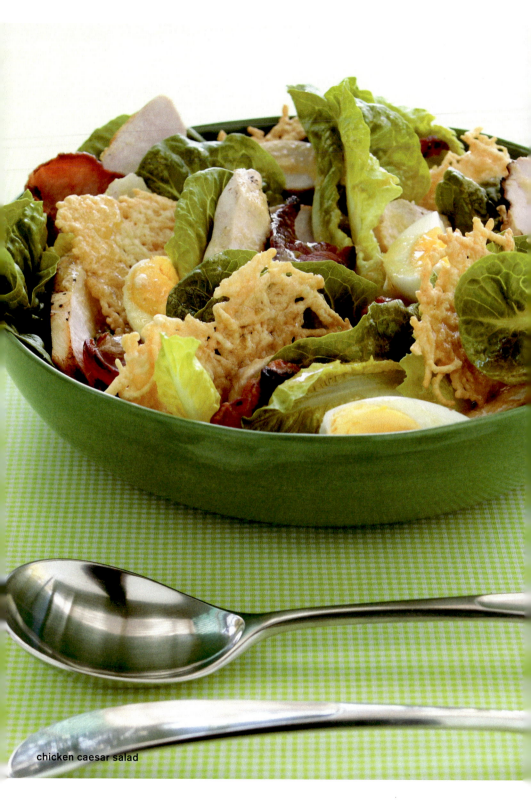
chicken caesar salad

CHICKEN CAESAR SALAD

1 Preheat oven to 200°C (400°F/Gas 6). Line 2 baking trays with baking paper.
2 Sprinkle the parmesan onto the prepared trays in triangle shapes. Bake for 10 minutes or until crisp and golden. Allow to cool on the trays.
3 Lightly spray a chargrill pan with olive oil spray and cook the chicken over medium heat for 15 minutes or until tender. Set aside for 10 minutes before slicing.
4 Process the garlic and salt in a food processor. Add the anchovies, lemon juice and Worcestershire. With the motor running, add the oil a drop at a time.
5 Toss the lettuce leaves with the dressing and divide among 4 serving bowls. Top with the bacon, eggs, chicken and parmesan triangles. Serves 4

per serve | fat 51.2 g | saturated fat 13.9 g | protein 51.1 g | carbohydrate 1.7 g | fibre 1.4 g | cholesterol 244 mg | energy 2807 kJ (668 Cal) | gi < 20 ▼ low

- 1 cup (100 g/3⅓ oz) finely grated parmesan cheese
- olive oil spray
- 500 g (1 lb) skinless chicken breasts
- 4 cloves garlic, chopped
- ½ teaspoon salt
- 2 anchovy fillets
- 2 teaspoons lemon juice
- 1 teaspoon gluten-free Worcestershire sauce
- ½ cup (125 ml/4 fl oz) extra virgin olive oil
- 2 baby cos lettuces
- 200 g (6½ oz) trimmed bacon, grilled until crisp
- 2 hard-boiled eggs, quartered

SWEET POTATO & SALMON PATTIES

1 Cook the rice in a pan of boiling water for 15 minutes or until soft. Drain well.
2 Cook the sweet potato in a large pan of boiling water for 20 minutes or until soft. Drain well and mash.
3 Combine the rice, sweet potato, salmon, spring onions, seeds, almond meal, lemon zest and parsley and season. Shape the mixture into 8 flat patties, roll in the cornflakes and refrigerate for 15 minutes.
4 Preheat oven to 200°C (400°F/Gas 6).
5 Place the patties on a non-stick baking tray and spray with olive oil spray. Bake for 20 minutes or until golden and heated through. Serve with gluten-free sweet chilli sauce and a green salad. Makes 8

per ball | fat 7.3 g | saturated fat 1.4 g | protein 11 g | carbohydrate 21.2 g | fibre 2.2 g | cholesterol 25 mg | energy 831 kJ (198 Cal) | gi 60 ◆ med

- ½ cup (75 g/2½ oz) brown rice
- 500 g (1 lb) orange sweet potato, peeled and chopped
- 400 g (13 oz) can red salmon in brine, drained
- 3 spring onions (scallions), sliced
- 3 tablespoons sunflower seeds
- 2 tablespoons almond meal
- 1 teaspoon lemon zest
- 2 tablespoons chopped fresh parsley
- salt and pepper
- 1½ cups (45 g/1½ oz) gluten-free cornflakes
- olive oil spray

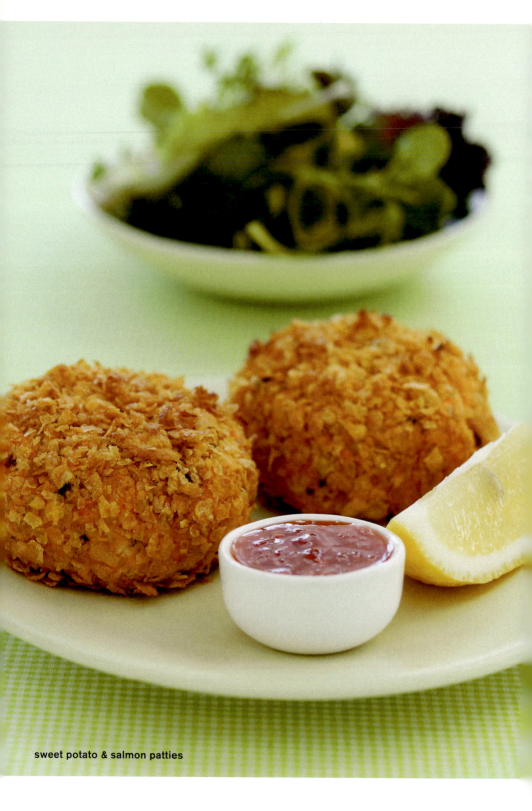

sweet potato & salmon patties

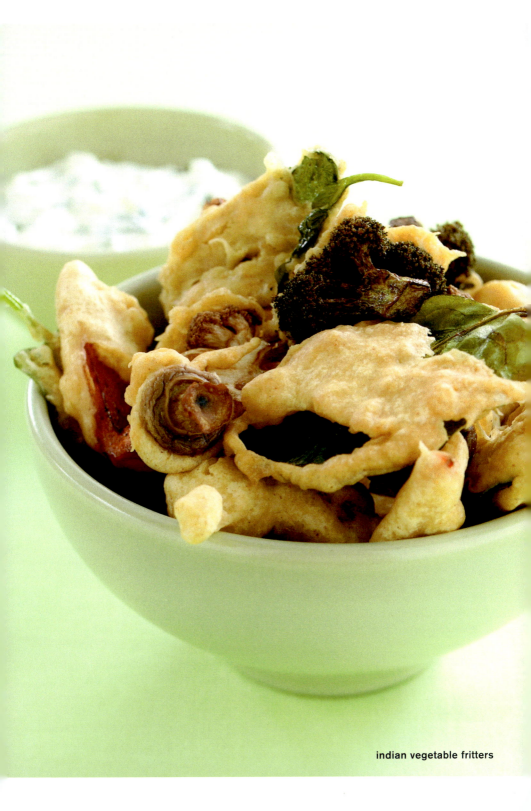

indian vegetable fritters

INDIAN VEGETABLE FRITTERS

225 g (7 oz) chickpea flour (besan)
1 teaspoon salt
1 teaspoon ground cumin
1 teaspoon ground coriander
½ teaspoon chilli powder
300 ml (10 fl oz) soda water
peanut oil for deep frying
300 g (10 oz) cauliflower, cut into florets
200 g (6½ oz) broccoli, cut into florets
1 medium red capsicum (bell pepper), sliced
100 g (3⅓ oz) button mushrooms
20 g (¾ oz) baby English spinach
200 g (6½ oz) low-fat plain yoghurt
1 tablespoon chopped fresh mint
1 clove garlic, crushed

1 Sift the chickpea flour, salt, cumin, coriander and chilli powder into a bowl. Slowly whisk in the soda water to form a smooth batter.
2 Heat the oil in a large wok or heavy-based pan over medium heat for 5 minutes or until the oil starts to move. Stand a wooden chopstick in the oil. If the oil bubbles around the chopstick, it is ready.
3 Dip the vegetables into the batter, then carefully lower into the oil. Do not overcrowd the oil. You may need to cook a few batches at a time. Cook for 5 minutes or until the vegetables are crisp and golden. Drain on absorbent paper.
4 Put the yoghurt, mint and garlic into a bowl and mix to combine. Serve with the hot fritters. Serves 4

per serve | fat 6.8 g | saturated fat 3.5 g | protein 21.2 g | carbohydrate 39 g | fibre 11.1 g | cholesterol 3 mg | energy 1334 kJ (318 Cal) | gi 43 ▼ low

* The batter may also be used to coat other foods that are to be deep fried.

BEEF YAKITORI

500 g (1 lb) lean rump steak, thinly sliced
8 spring onions (scallions), cut into 5 cm (2 in) pieces
1 medium red capsicum (bell pepper), cut into cubes
100 g (3⅓ oz) shiitake mushrooms
⅓ cup (80 ml/2⅔ fl oz) gluten-free tamari
⅓ cup (80 ml/2⅔ fl oz) mirin
2 tablespoons sugar

1 Soak 12 bamboo skewers in water for 15 minutes to prevent them from burning on the barbecue.
2 Thread the beef, spring onions, capsicum and mushrooms onto the skewers.
3 Put the tamari, mirin and sugar into a pan and stir over low heat until the sugar has dissolved. Bring to the boil, then reduce the heat and simmer for 5 minutes or until reduced by half.
4 Cook the beef skewers on a barbecue for 3 minutes, then baste generously with the yakitori sauce. Cook for another 3 minutes or until the beef is tender. Makes 12

per skewer | fat 2 g | saturated fat 0.8 g | protein 10 g | carbohydrate 3.9 g | fibre 0.5 g | cholesterol 27 mg | energy 313 kJ (74 Cal) | gi 45 ▼ low

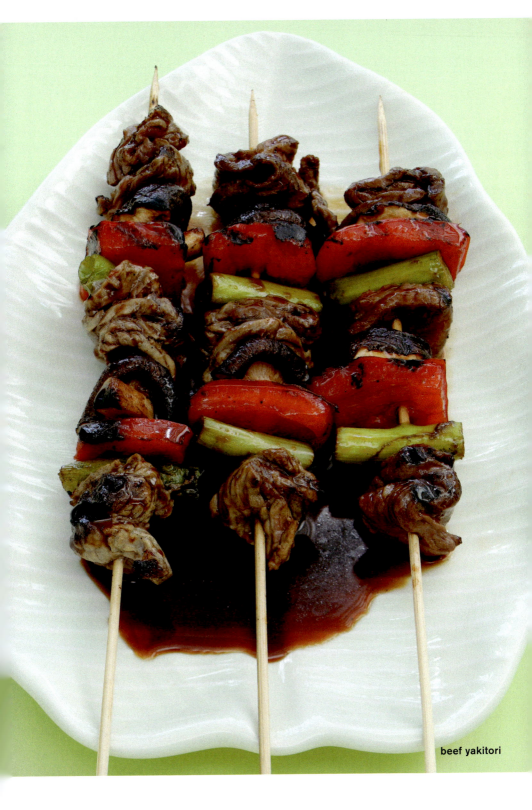

beef yakitori

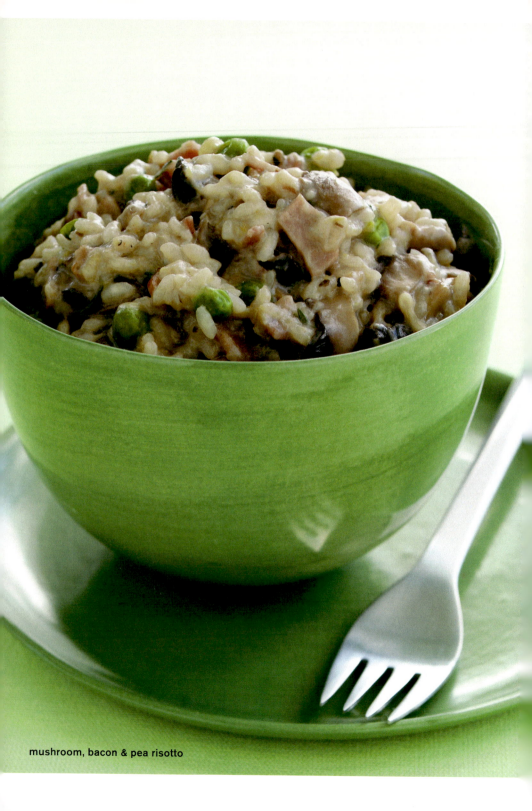

mushroom, bacon & pea risotto

MUSHROOM, BACON & PEA RISOTTO

1 Put the chicken stock and water into a pan and bring to the boil. Reduce the heat and keep at simmering point.
2 Heat the oil in a large pan over medium heat, add the leeks and garlic and cook for 5 minutes or until the leeks are soft and golden.
3 Add the rice and cook, stirring, for 2 minutes or until translucent. Add the bacon and mushrooms and cook for 3 minutes or until the mushrooms start to soften.
4 Add ½ cup (125 ml/4 fl oz) of the simmering stock and stir until most of the liquid has been absorbed. Continue adding the stock ½ cup (125 ml/4 fl oz) at a time until all the liquid has been absorbed and the rice is soft and creamy. Add the peas with the last of the stock.
5 Remove from the heat, stir in the evaporated milk, parmesan and herbs and beat until creamy. Season with salt and pepper. Serves 6

per serve | fat 8.4 g | saturated fat 3.4 g | protein 19.9 g | carbohydrate 48.3 g | fibre 4.1 g | cholesterol 28 mg | energy 1465 kJ (349 Cal) | gi 59 ◆ med

* Any leftover risotto can be shaped into balls, tossed in gluten-free all-purpose crumbs and fried until golden. Transfer to the oven to heat through.

- 3 cups (750 ml/24 fl oz) gluten-free chicken stock made from a stock cube
- 1 cup (250 ml/8 fl oz) water
- 2 teaspoons olive oil
- 2 medium leeks, sliced
- 2 cloves garlic, crushed
- 1½ cups (305 g/10 oz) arborio rice
- 200 g (6½ oz) trimmed bacon, chopped
- 300 g (10 oz) field mushrooms, sliced
- 1 cup (150 g/5 oz) fresh or frozen peas
- ½ cup (125 ml/4 fl oz) reduced-fat evaporated milk
- ½ cup (50 g/1⅔ oz) finely grated parmesan cheese
- 2 tablespoons chopped fresh herbs (parsley, thyme, chives)
- salt and pepper

DESSERT

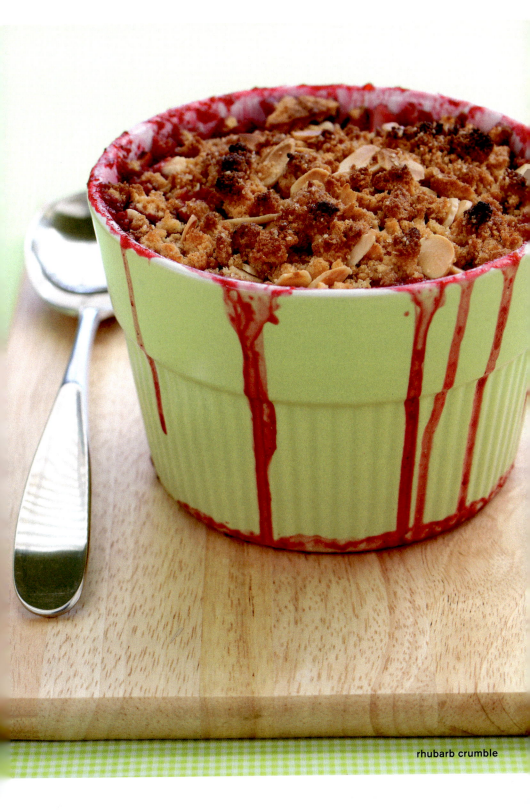

rhubarb crumble

RHUBARB CRUMBLE

1 kg (2 lb) rhubarb, cut into 3 cm (1¼ in) pieces
¼ cup (60 ml/2 fl oz) water
½ cup (115 g/3⅔ oz) firmly packed brown sugar
1 vanilla bean, halved lengthwise
180 g (6 oz) gluten-free coconut biscuits, roughly crushed
50 g (1⅔ oz) butter or canola margarine, chopped
50 g (1⅔ oz) flaked almonds
2 tablespoons demerara sugar
½ teaspoon mixed spice

1 Preheat oven to 200°C (400°F/Gas 6).
2 Put the rhubarb, water, brown sugar and vanilla bean into a pan, cover and cook over medium heat for 5-10 minutes or until the rhubarb is just soft. Remove the vanilla bean. Transfer the mixture to a 6 cup (1.5 litre/48 fl oz) capacity ovenproof dish.
3 Put half the crushed coconut biscuits into a bowl and rub in the butter or margarine until the mixture resembles fine breadcrumbs. Add the remaining biscuits, flaked almonds, sugar and mixed spice.
4 Spoon the biscuit mixture over the rhubarb. Bake the crumble for 15-20 minutes or until the topping is crisp and golden. Serves 6

per serve | fat 17.1 g | saturated fat 7.1 g | protein 5 g | carbohydrate 50.6 g | fibre 4.8 g | cholesterol 12 mg | energy 1537 kJ (366 Cal) | gi 49 ▼ low

MANGO COCONUT SAGO PUDDING

½ cup (95 g/3 oz) sago
2 cups (500 ml/16 fl oz) mango puree
2 cups (500 ml/16 fl oz) water
zest of 1 lime
1 vanilla bean, halved lengthwise
3 tablespoons brown sugar
½ cup (125 ml/4 fl oz) coconut cream
1 teaspoon gelatin

1 Put the sago, mango puree, water, lime zest, vanilla bean and 2 tablespoons of the brown sugar into a pan. Stir over low heat until the sugar has dissolved. Bring to the boil, then reduce the heat to medium and cook, stirring, for 10 minutes or until the sago is clear and soft. Remove the vanilla bean. Divide the sago among 4 serving glasses.
2 Put the coconut cream, gelatin and remaining sugar into a pan and stir over low heat for 5 minutes or until the sugar and gelatin have dissolved.
3 Pour the coconut mixture onto the sago and refrigerate for 4 hours or until the coconut jelly is set. Serves 4

per serve | fat 6.9 g | saturated fat 5.7 g | protein 2.8 g | carbohydrate 48.4 g | fibre 3 g | cholesterol 0 mg | energy 1135 kJ (270 Cal) | gi 52 ▼ low

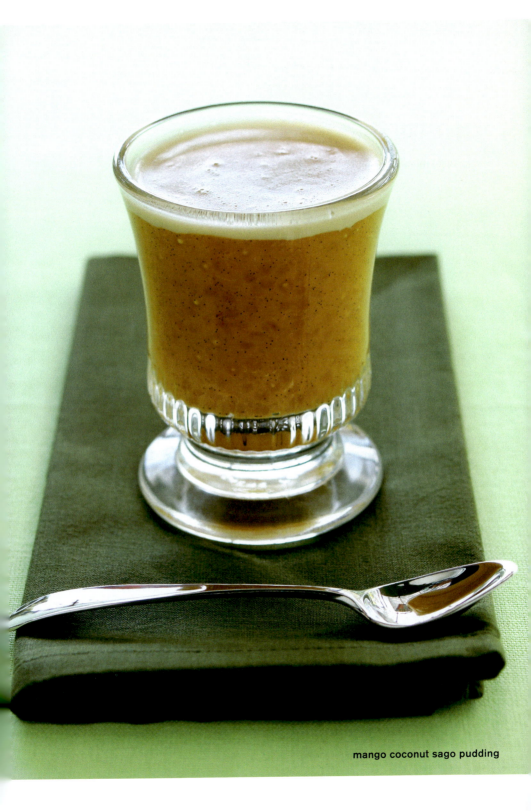

mango coconut sago pudding

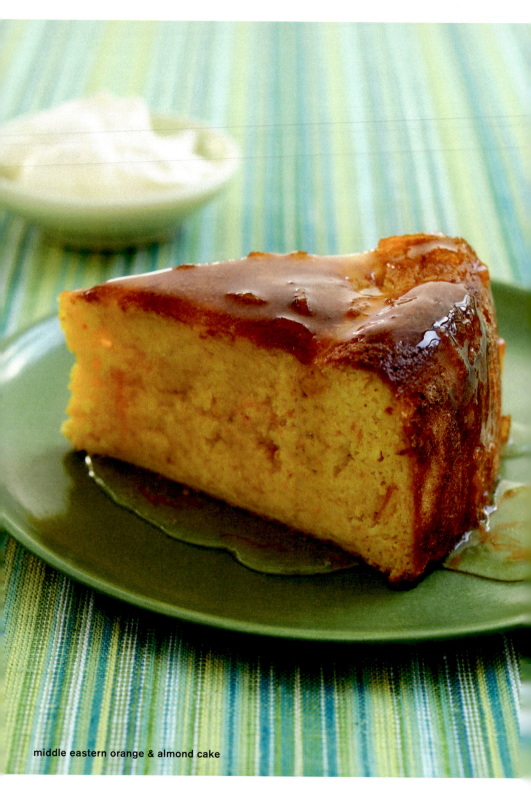

middle eastern orange & almond cake

MIDDLE EASTERN ORANGE & ALMOND CAKE

1 Wash the oranges and scrub the skins. Put the whole oranges into a pan, cover with water and boil for 2 hours or until very soft. Drain and leave to cool.
2 Preheat oven to 190°C (375°F/Gas 5). Line a 22 cm (9 in) spring form tin with baking paper.
3 Put the cooled oranges into a food processor or blender and blend until smooth.
4 Whisk the eggs in a large bowl. Add the pureed oranges, almond meal and 1 cup (250 g/8 oz) of the sugar and mix to combine. Spoon the mixture into the prepared tin and bake for 1¼ hours or until a skewer comes out clean when inserted into the center. Leave to cool in the tin for 5 minutes.
5 Put the remaining sugar into a pan with the water and orange zest and stir over low heat until the sugar has dissolved. Bring to the boil and cook over high heat for 5 minutes or until syrupy. Serve wedges of the cake with the sauce drizzled over the top. Serves 8

2 large navel oranges
6 eggs
2½ cups (250 g/8 oz) almond meal
1½ cups (375 g/12 oz) caster sugar
½ cup (125 ml/4 fl oz) water
zest of 1 orange

per serve | fat 21.1 g | saturated fat 2.3 g | protein 11.6 g | carbohydrate 52.6 g | fibre 3.8 g | cholesterol 141 mg | energy 1854 kJ (441 Cal) | gi 58 ◆ med

WHITE CHOCOLATE RASPBERRY CHEESECAKE

125 g (4 oz) gluten-free rice cookies, roughly crushed
½ cup (50 g/1⅔ oz) almond meal
60 g (2 oz) butter or reduced-fat margarine, melted
500 g (1 lb) white chocolate, chopped
1 cup (250 ml/8 fl oz) cream
500 g (1 lb) cream cheese, softened and chopped*
½ cup (125 g/4 oz) caster sugar
200 g (6½ oz) fresh or frozen raspberries

1 Lightly grease and line a 20 cm (8 in) spring form tin.
2 Put the rice cookies and almond meal into a food processor and process until finely crushed.
3 Transfer the mixture to a bowl and stir in the butter or margarine. Press into the base of the tin and refrigerate for 30 minutes or until firm.
4 Put the white chocolate and cream into a pan and cook, stirring, over low heat for 5 minutes or until the chocolate has melted and the mixture is smooth. Remove from the heat and set aside to cool slightly.
5 Beat the cream cheese and sugar until light and fluffy. Fold through the white chocolate mixture. Pour the mixture into the tin and chill overnight or until firm.
6 Serve the cheesecake topped with the raspberries.
Serves 12

per serve | fat 45.6 g | saturated fat 26.5 g | protein 8.8 g | carbohydrate 41.8 g | fibre 1.7 g | cholesterol 86 mg | energy 2523 kJ (600 Cal) | gi 47 ▼ low

* You can make this cheesecake using reduced-fat cream cheese; however, the texture will be much softer.

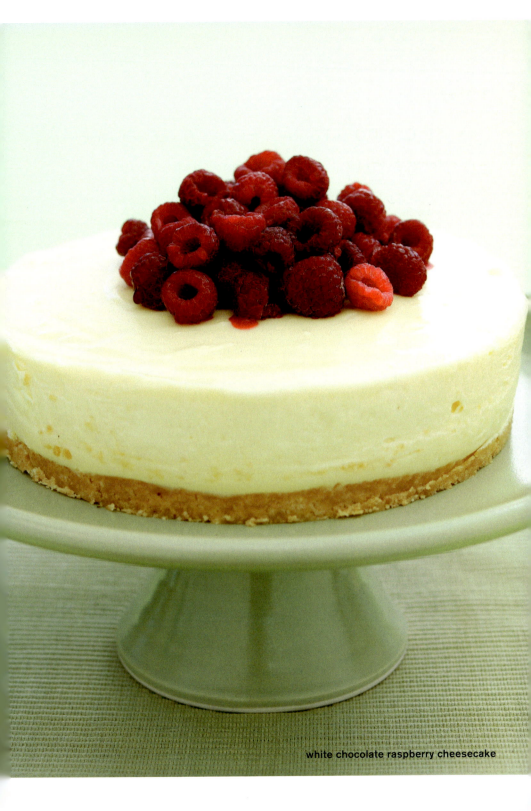

white chocolate raspberry cheesecake

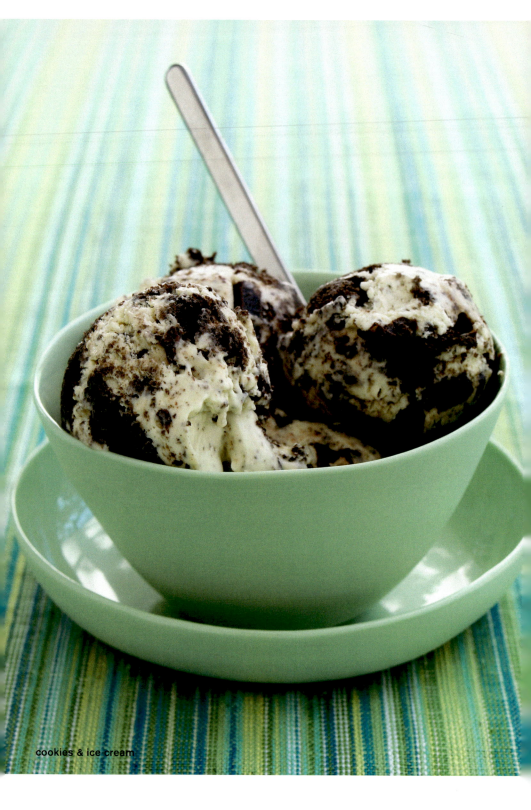

cookies & ice cream

COOKIES & ICE CREAM

1 Put the cream and condensed milk into a bowl and beat until thick and creamy.
2 Fold the chocolate biscuits and dark chocolate through the cream mixture.
3 Pour the mixture into an 8 cup (2 litre/64 fl oz) ice cream container and freeze until firm. Makes 2 litres
per ½ cup (125 ml/4 fl oz) | fat 17.9 g | saturated fat 5.7 g | protein 3.7 g | carbohydrate 13.6 g | fibre 1 g | cholesterol 47 mg | energy 456 kJ (109 Cal) | gi 51 ▼ low

600 ml (20 fl oz) thickened cream
395 g (13 oz) can skim sweetened condensed milk
180 g (6 oz) gluten-free chocolate biscuits, roughly crushed
100 g (3⅓ oz) dark chocolate, roughly chopped

CREPES WITH BLUEBERRIES

1 Place the blueberries, sugar and 300 ml (10 fl oz) of the water into a pan and cook over low heat for 5 minutes or until the sugar has dissolved.
2 Mix the arrowroot with the remaining water and stir into the blueberries. Simmer, stirring, until the sauce thickens. Cover and set aside until ready to serve.
3 Sift the flour into a bowl, stir in the sugar and make a well in the center. Whisk together the butter or margarine, eggs and milk. Pour into the well and mix until the batter is smooth.
4 Lightly grease a small non-stick fry pan with canola oil spray. Pour 2-3 tablespoons of the batter into the pan and tilt to cover the base with the batter. Cook over medium heat for 2 minutes or until the crepe is golden on the underside. Turn the crepe over and cook the other side until golden. Keep warm while you cook the remaining batter. Serve the crepes with the blueberries. Serves 4
per serve | fat 7.1 g | saturated fat 2.4 g | protein 7 g | carbohydrate 43.5 g | fibre 2.5 g | cholesterol 102 mg | energy 1113 kJ (265 Cal) | gi 52 ▼ low

300 g (10 oz) fresh blueberries
¼ cup (60 g/2 oz) caster sugar
320 ml (10⅔ fl oz) water
2 teaspoons arrowroot
70 g (2¼ oz) gluten-free all-purpose flour pre mix
1 tablespoon caster sugar
20 g (¾ oz) butter or canola margarine, melted
2 eggs
¾ cup (185 ml/6 fl oz) skim or no-fat milk
canola oil spray

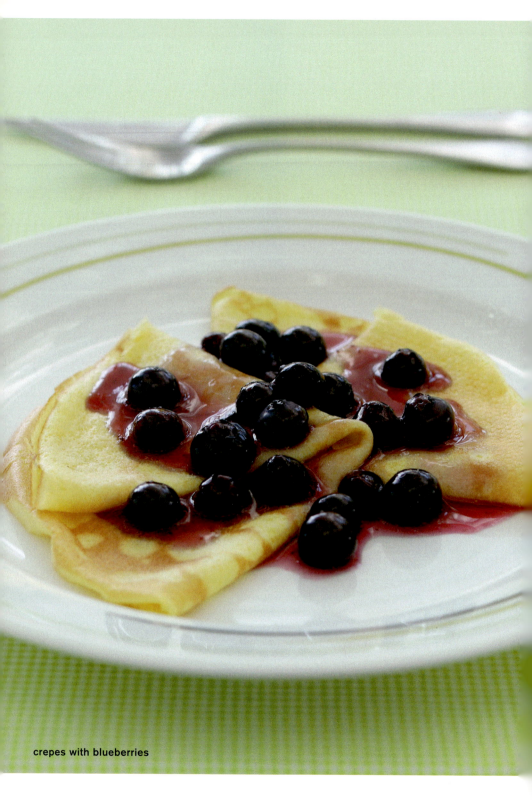
crepes with blueberries

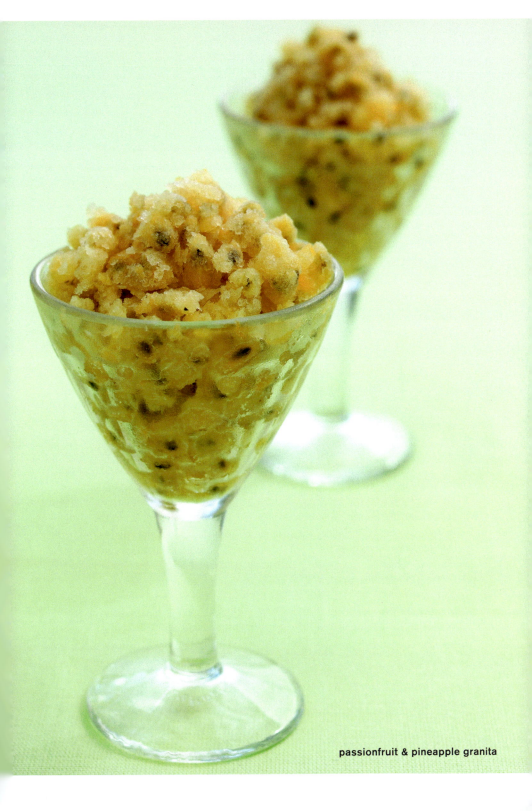
passionfruit & pineapple granita

PASSIONFRUIT & PINEAPPLE GRANITA

300 ml (10 fl oz) passionfruit pulp
300 ml (10 fl oz) unsweetened pineapple juice
¼ cup (60 ml/2 fl oz) lime juice
½ cup (125 g/4 oz) caster sugar

1 Put the passionfruit pulp, pineapple juice, lime juice and sugar into a bowl and mix to combine.
2 Pour the mixture into a shallow metal container, cover and freeze for 2 hours or until the edges are just frozen.
3 Scrape the mixture with a fork to break up the ice crystals, then return to the freezer for 1 hour. Repeat the scraping and freezing 5 times over the next 3-4 hours or until the ice crystals are even in size.
4 Scrape the granita with a fork to break it up. Serve the granita in glasses. Serves 6

per serve | fat 0.2 g | saturated fat 0 g | protein 1.8 g | carbohydrate 29.2 g | fibre 7 g | cholesterol 0 mg | energy 591 kJ (141 Cal) | gi 53 ▼ low

STICKY DATE & POLENTA PUDDINGS

⅔ cup (170 ml/5⅔ fl oz) golden syrup
1 cup (185 g/6 oz) sliced pitted fresh dates
4 cups (1 litre/32 fl oz) milk
⅓ cup (80 g/2⅔ oz) caster sugar
40 g (1⅓ oz) butter or canola margarine, melted
¾ cup (110 g/3½ oz) fine polenta (cornmeal)
½ cup (125 ml/4 fl oz) reduced-fat cream

1 Preheat oven to 160°C (315°F/Gas 2-3). Lightly grease 6 x 1 cup (250 ml/8 fl oz) capacity ramekins.
2 Put the golden syrup and dates into a pan over medium heat and simmer for 5 minutes or until the dates have softened. Divide the dates and golden syrup among the prepared ramekins.
3 Heat the milk, sugar and butter or margarine in a pan over medium heat until just simmering. Whisk in the polenta and cook, stirring constantly, for 15 minutes or until the polenta is thick and creamy. Remove from the heat and stir in the cream.
4 Spoon the mixture into the ramekins and smooth the surface. Bake for 25 minutes or until set. Invert the puddings onto plates and serve with fresh cream. Serves 6

per serve | fat 17.2 g | saturated fat 10.1 g | protein 8.2 g | carbohydrate 72.7 g | fibre 2 g | cholesterol 47 mg | energy 1969 kJ (469 Cal) | gi 47 ▼ low

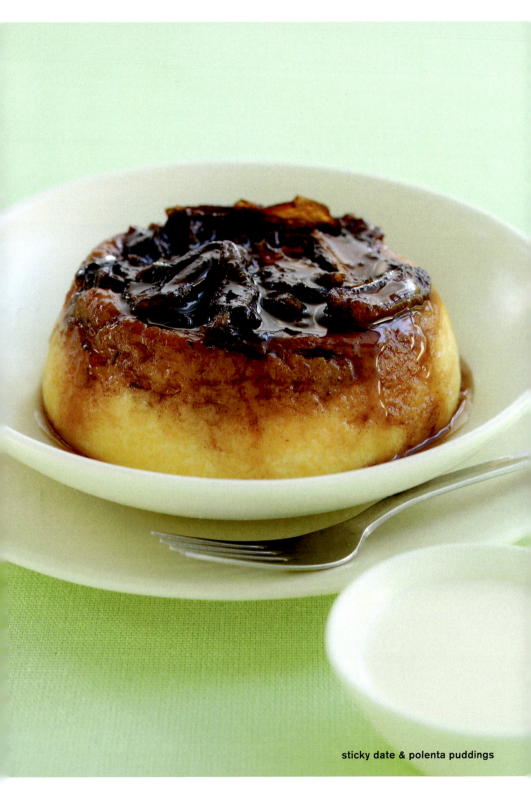

sticky date & polenta puddings

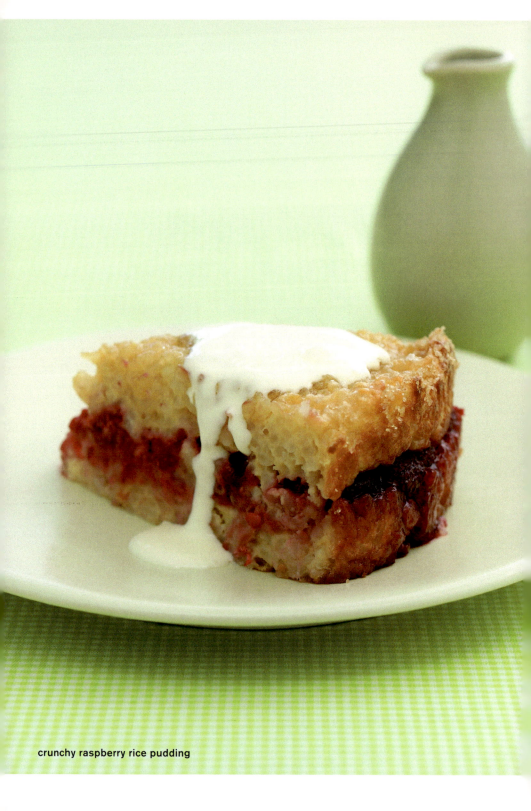

crunchy raspberry rice pudding

CRUNCHY RASPBERRY RICE PUDDING

1 Preheat oven to 180°C (350°F/Gas 4). Lightly grease an 18 cm (7 in) spring form tin.
2 Put the milk and rice into a pan and bring slowly to the boil. Reduce the heat to low, cover and simmer, stirring occasionally, for 30 minutes or until the rice is soft.
3 Add the brown sugar, butter or margarine and lemon zest and mix well to combine. Set aside to cool.
4 Sprinkle the side of the prepared tin with the demerara sugar. Reserve any remaining sugar.
5 Add the beaten eggs to the cooled rice mixture and mix well to combine. Spoon half of the mixture into the prepared tin, sprinkle with the raspberries and then top with the remaining rice mixture. Sprinkle with any remaining demerara sugar.
6 Bake for 40 minutes or until the top is golden brown and has formed a crust. Transfer to a rack and leave to cool slightly before serving. Serves 8

per serve | fat 10.5 g | saturated fat 5.2 g | protein 7 g | carbohydrate 40.8 g | fibre 1.7 | cholesterol 69 mg | energy 1200 kJ (286 Cal) | gi 63 ◆ med

* If you wish to lower the GI of this recipe, replace the short-grain rice with basmati rice or Doongara (CleverRice™).

3 cups (750 ml/24 fl oz) milk
1 cup (220 g/7 oz) short-grain rice
⅓ cup (80 g/2⅔ oz) firmly packed brown sugar
60 g (2 oz) butter or canola margarine, melted
zest of 1 lemon
2 tablespoons demerara sugar
2 eggs, lightly beaten
200 g (6½ oz) fresh or frozen raspberries

VANILLA & SAFFRON RICE SOUFFLES

3 cups (750 ml/24 fl oz) skim or no-fat milk
75 g (2½ oz) long-grain rice
2 teaspoons lemon zest
1 vanilla bean, halved lengthwise
pinch saffron threads
1 egg white
2 tablespoons caster sugar

1 Put the milk, rice, lemon zest, vanilla bean and saffron into a pan and slowly bring to the boil. Cook over low-medium heat, stirring regularly, for 45 minutes or until the rice is soft and creamy. Remove from the heat and discard the vanilla bean. Transfer the rice to a bowl, cover with plastic wrap and set aside to cool.

2 Preheat oven to 180°C (350°F/Gas 4). Lightly brush 4 x ½ cup (125 ml/4 fl oz) capacity ramekins with melted butter.

3 Whisk the egg white in a clean, dry bowl until stiff peaks form. Gradually add the sugar and beat until stiff and glossy.

4 Fold the egg white mixture through the rice mixture. Spoon into the prepared ramekins and bake for 20-25 minutes or until the souffles are puffed and golden. Serves 4

per serve | fat 0.3 g | saturated fat 0.2 g | protein 9.1 g | carbohydrate 33 g | fibre 0.2 g | cholesterol 6 mg | energy 711 kJ (169 Cal) | gi 49 ▼ low

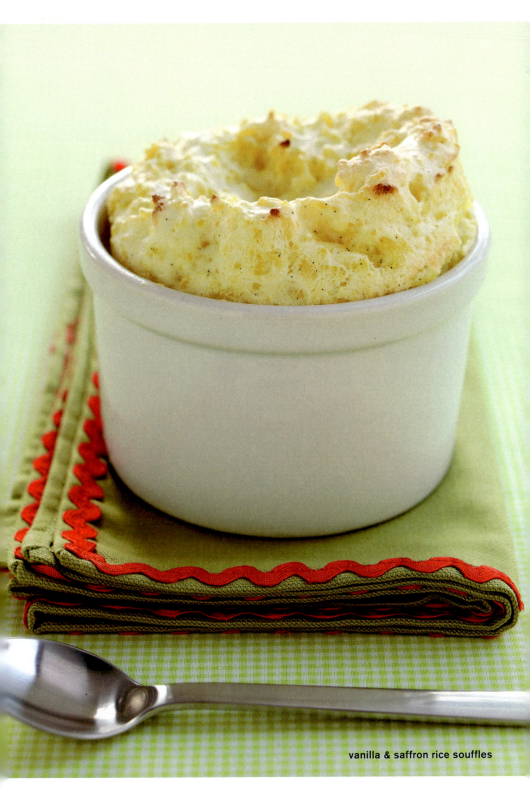

vanilla & saffron rice souffles

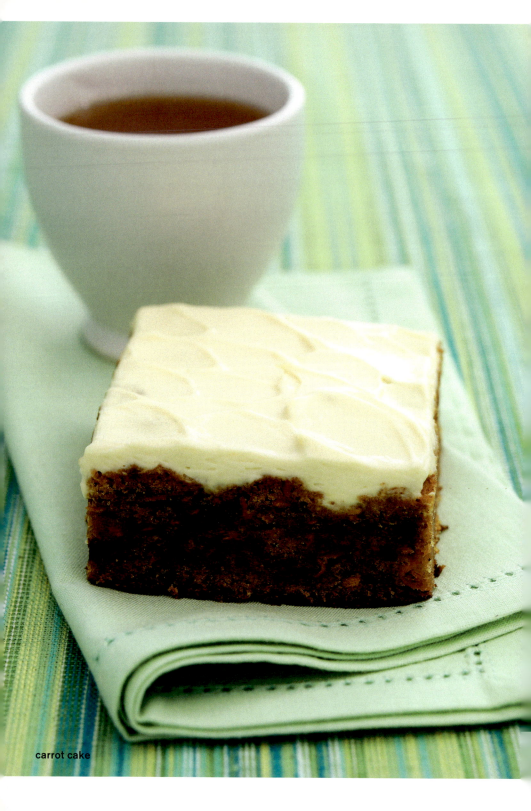

carrot cake

CARROT CAKE

1 Preheat oven to 180°C (350°F/Gas 4). Lightly grease a 23 cm (9 in) square cake tin and line the base with baking paper.
2 Sift the flour, baking powder, cinnamon and mixed spice into a bowl and stir in the baby rice cereal.
3 Whisk together the oil, sugar, eggs and golden syrup. Stir into the dry ingredients and mix well to combine. Stir in the grated carrot and walnuts.
4 Spoon the mixture into the prepared tin and bake for 1 hour 10 minutes or until a skewer comes out clean when inserted into the center. Allow to cool in the tin for 15 minutes before turning out on a wire rack to cool completely.
5 To make the icing, beat the mascarpone cheese, yoghurt and maple syrup until smooth. Spread over the cold cake. Serves 12

per serve | fat 17.6 g | saturated fat 4.1 g | protein 5.7 g | carbohydrate 41.5 g | fibre 2.1 g | cholesterol 73 mg | energy 1450 kJ (345 Cal) | gi 60 ◆ med

- 1½ cups (180 g/6 oz) gluten-free self-raising flour
- 2 teaspoons gluten-free baking powder
- 2 teaspoons ground cinnamon
- 1 teaspoon mixed spice
- 2½ cups (150 g/5 oz) baby rice cereal
- ½ cup (125 ml/4 fl oz) olive oil
- 1 cup (185 g/6 oz) lightly packed brown sugar
- 4 eggs, lightly beaten
- ¼ cup (60 ml/2 fl oz) golden syrup
- 2½ cups (390 g/12½ oz) grated carrot
- ½ cup (50 g/1⅔ oz) walnuts, roughly chopped
- 3 tablespoons mascarpone cheese
- 3 tablespoons plain yoghurt
- 2 teaspoons maple syrup

BREADS & BAKING

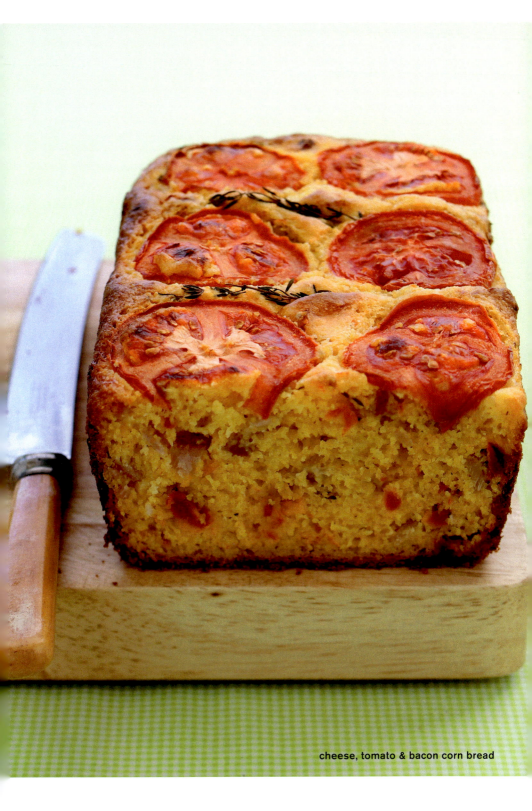

cheese, tomato & bacon corn bread

CHEESE, TOMATO & BACON CORN BREAD

1¼ cups (150 g/5 oz) gluten-free self-raising flour
1 tablespoon caster sugar
2 teaspoons gluten-free baking powder
1 teaspoon salt
¾ cup (110 g/3½ oz) fine polenta (cornmeal)
½ cup (60 g/2 oz) grated cheddar cheese
1 teaspoon chopped fresh thyme
100 g (3⅓ oz) semi-dried tomatoes, finely chopped
100 g (3⅓ oz) trimmed bacon, chopped
2 eggs, lightly beaten
1 cup (250 ml/8 fl oz) buttermilk
⅓ cup (80 ml/2⅔ fl oz) olive oil
1 medium tomato, sliced
3 fresh thyme sprigs

1 Preheat oven to 180°C (350°F/Gas 4). Line a 20 cm x 10 cm (8 in x 4 in) loaf tin with baking paper.
2 Sift the flour, sugar, baking powder and salt into a bowl. Stir in the polenta, cheese, thyme, tomatoes and bacon and make a well in the center.
3 Whisk together the eggs, buttermilk and oil, pour into the well and mix until well combined.
4 Spoon the mixture into the prepared tin and decorate the top with the tomato slices and thyme sprigs. Bake for 45 minutes or until a skewer comes out clean when inserted into the center. Store the corn bread wrapped in plastic in an airtight container for up to 2 days. It is delicious toasted. Serves 8
per serve | fat 15.9 g | saturated fat 4.2 g | protein 10.5 g | carbohydrate 26.5 g | fibre 2.2 g | cholesterol 65 mg | energy 1234 kJ (294 Cal) | gi 54 ▼ low

FLOURLESS FRUIT & NUT COOKIES

½ cup (80 g/2⅔ oz) raw unsalted peanuts, roughly chopped
½ cup (80 g/2⅔ oz) hazelnuts, toasted and roughly chopped
300 g (10 oz) shredded coconut
125 g (4 oz) dried apricots, roughly chopped
50 g (1⅔ oz) sultanas
125 g (4 oz) dark chocolate, roughly chopped
500 g (1 lb) sweetened condensed milk

1 Preheat oven to 160°C (315°F/Gas 2-3). Line 2 baking trays with baking paper.
2 Put the nuts, coconut, apricots, sultanas and chocolate into a bowl and mix to combine. Add the condensed milk and mix well.
3 Drop tablespoons of the nut mixture onto the prepared trays, allowing room for spreading. Bake for 20 minutes or until the cookies are crisp and golden brown. Makes 20
per cookie | fat 17.5 g | saturated fat 12.2 g | protein 4.9 g | carbohydrate 23.5 g | fibre 3.8 g | cholesterol 9 mg | energy 1141 kJ (272 Cal) | gi 50 ▼ low

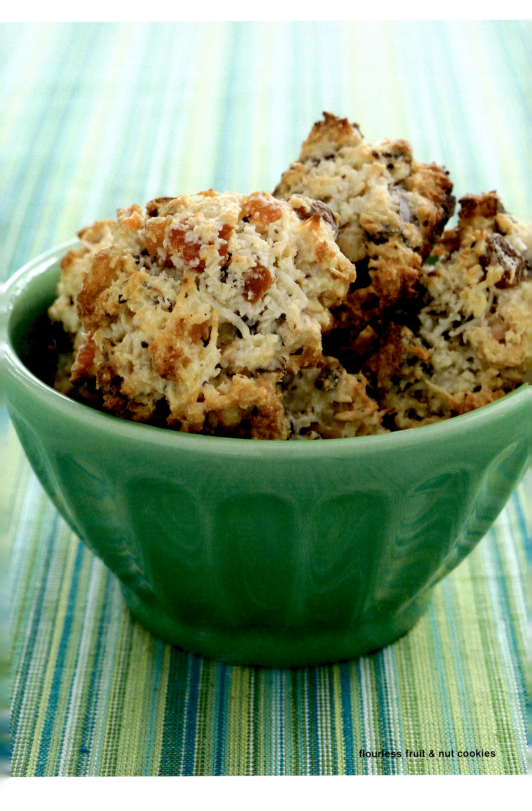

flourless fruit & nut cookies

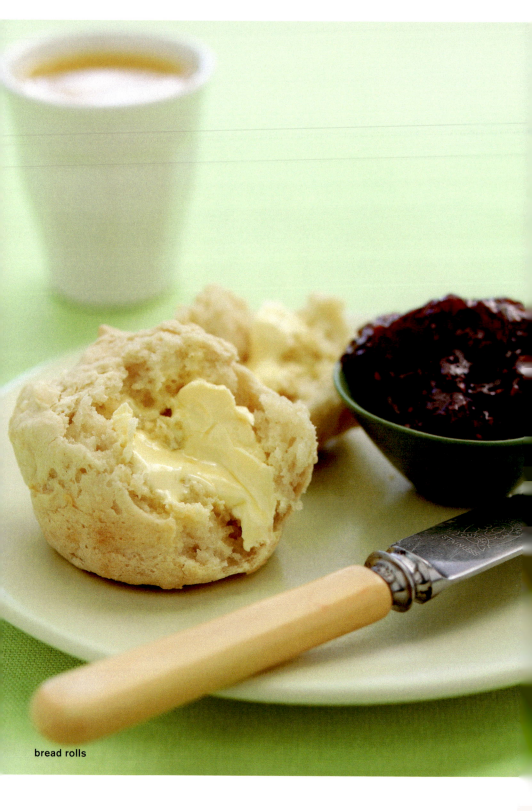

bread rolls

BREAD ROLLS

1 Preheat oven to 230°C (450°F/Gas 8). Lightly grease a 12 x ½ cup (125 ml/4 fl oz) capacity non-stick muffin pan.
2 Sift the flour, salt and sugar into a bowl, stir in the yeast and cheese and make a well in the center.
3 Whisk together the egg, water and oil, pour into the well and stir into the dry ingredients. Mix well with electric beaters for 5 minutes.
4 Spoon the mixture into the muffin holes, cover with lightly oiled plastic wrap and set aside to rise in a warm place for 45 minutes.
5 Remove the plastic wrap. Sprinkle the rolls with sesame seeds and bake for 25 minutes. Leave to cool in the pan for 5 minutes before transferring to a wire rack to cool. These dense bread rolls are best eaten on the day they are baked. They can also be frozen and reheated in the microwave. Makes 12

per roll | fat 5.6 g | saturated fat 1.7 g | protein 5.3 g | carbohydrate 24.7 g | fibre 2.4 g | cholesterol 22 mg | energy 735 kJ (175 Cal) | gi 60 ◆ med

3½ cups (420 g/14 oz) gluten-free all-purpose flour pre mix
½ teaspoon salt
¼ teaspoon sugar
2 teaspoons dried yeast
½ cup (60 g/2 oz) grated cheddar cheese
1 egg, lightly beaten
1¾ cups (440 ml/14 fl oz) warm water
1 tablespoon olive oil
1 tablespoon sesame seeds (optional)

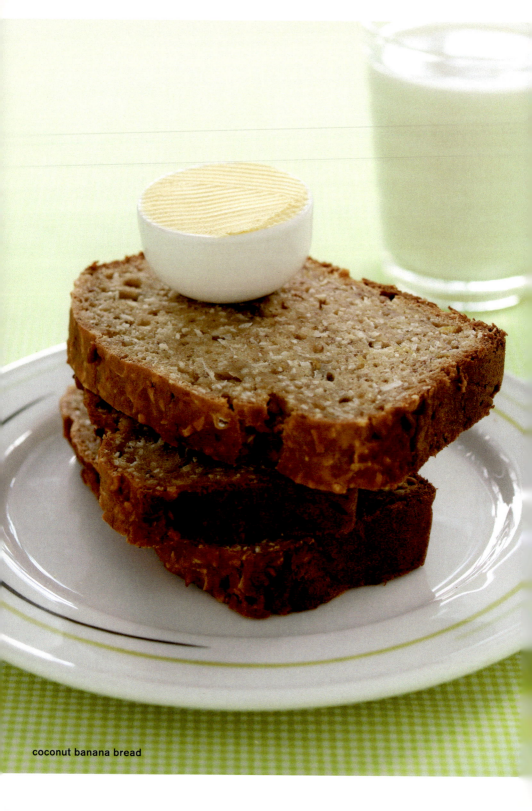

coconut banana bread

COCONUT BANANA BREAD

1 Preheat oven to 180°C (350°F/Gas 4). Line a 10 cm x 23 cm (4 in x 9 in) loaf tin with baking paper.
2 Sift the flour, baking powder and mixed spice into a bowl. Stir in the sugar and coconut and make a well in the center.
3 Whisk together the egg, egg whites, milk and butter or margarine, pour into the well and stir until just combined. Fold through the mashed bananas.
4 Spoon the mixture into the prepared tin and bake for 1 ¼ hours or until a skewer comes out clean when inserted into the center. Serve warm, cold or toasted, with your favourite spread. Serves 10
per serve | fat 12.3 g | saturated fat 8.7 g | protein 6.3 g | carbohydrate 51 g | fibre 4 g | cholesterol 32 mg | energy 1409 kJ (336 Cal) | gi 53 ▼ low

2 ½ cups (300 g/10 oz) gluten-free all-purpose flour pre mix
2 teaspoons gluten-free baking powder
2 teaspoons mixed spice
1 cup (230 g/7 ¼ oz) firmly packed brown sugar
100 g (3 ⅓ oz) shredded coconut
1 egg, lightly beaten
2 egg whites
300 ml (10 fl oz) reduced-fat milk
50 g (1 ⅔ oz) butter or canola margarine, melted
2 medium ripe bananas, mashed

PARMESAN & PEPPER SHORTBREAD

1 Preheat oven to 150°C (300°F/Gas 2). Line 2 baking trays with baking paper.
2 Put the parmesan, flour, rice cereal, salt and pepper into a bowl and mix to combine.
3 Beat the butter in a bowl until creamy. Add to the dry ingredients and mix in the oil and egg white to form a soft dough. Gather the dough together.
4 Roll out the dough to form a 20 cm (8 in) cylinder and refrigerate for 20 minutes.
5 Use a sharp knife to cut the dough into thin slices. Place on the prepared trays and bake for 20-25 minutes or until crisp and golden. Transfer to a wire rack to cool. Makes 20
per shortbread | fat 4.6 g | saturated fat 2.7 g | protein 2.1 g | carbohydrate 4.2 g | fibre 0.3 g | cholesterol 13 mg | energy 284 kJ (68 Cal) | gi 62 ◆ med

¾ cup (75 g/2 ½ oz) finely grated parmesan cheese
85 g (2 ¾ oz) gluten-free all-purpose flour pre mix
½ cup (30 g/1 oz) baby rice cereal
¼ teaspoon salt
½ teaspoon finely cracked black pepper
70 g (2 ¼ oz) butter, softened
2 teaspoons olive oil
1 egg white

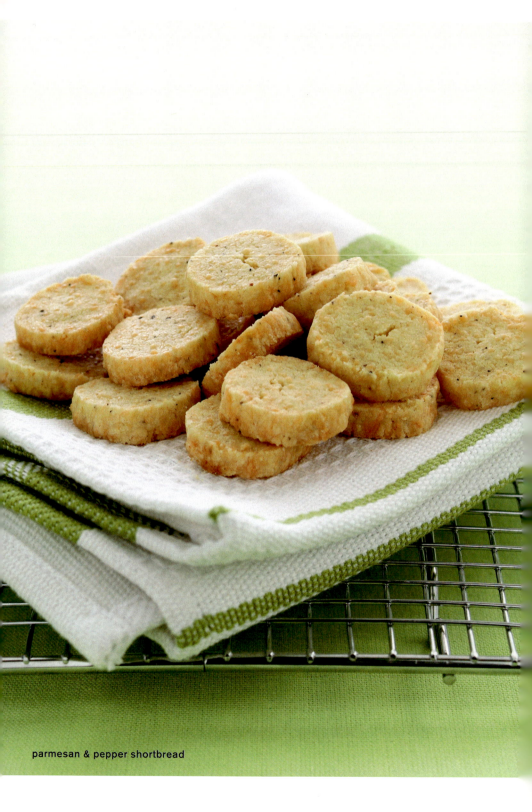

parmesan & pepper shortbread

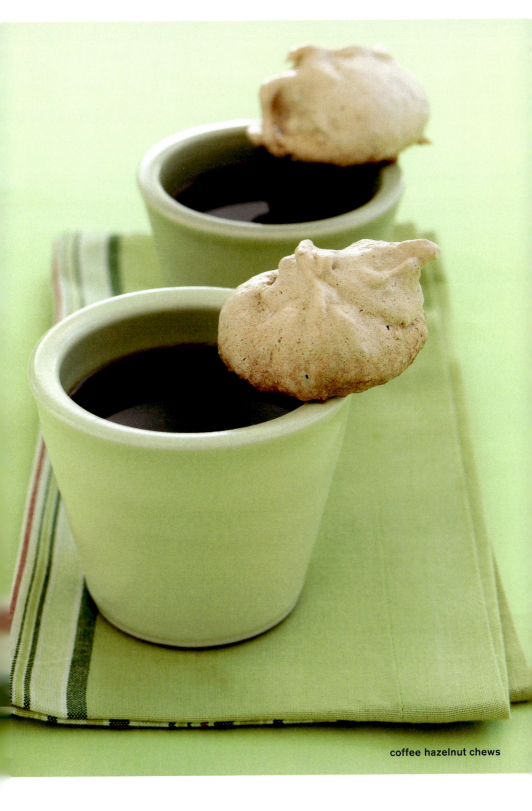

coffee hazelnut chews

COFFEE HAZELNUT CHEWS

5 egg whites
2/3 cup (170 g/5 2/3 oz) caster sugar
1/3 cup (80 g/2 2/3 oz) firmly packed brown sugar
1 teaspoon coffee essence (optional)
1/2 cup (95 g/3 oz) hazelnut meal

1 Preheat oven to 130°C (250°F/Gas 1). Line 2 baking trays with baking paper.
2 Whisk the egg whites in a clean, dry bowl until stiff peaks form. Gradually add the sugars and beat until stiff and glossy.
3 Fold the coffee essence and hazelnut meal through the egg white mixture. Drop heaped tablespoons of the mixture onto the prepared trays and bake for 45 minutes or until firm. Leave to cool in the oven with the door ajar. Makes 24

per chew | fat 2.4 g | saturated fat 0.1 g | protein 1.3 g | carbohydrate 10.5 g | fibre 0.4 g | cholesterol 0 mg | energy 284 kJ (68 Cal) | gi 60 ◆ med

DENSE FRUIT BREAD

200 g (6 1/2 oz) dried apricots, roughly chopped
200 g (6 1/2 oz) dried figs, roughly chopped
200 g (6 1/2 oz) pitted dried dates, roughly chopped
100 g (3 1/3 oz) raisins
2 cups (500 ml/16 fl oz) water
1 teaspoon bicarbonate of soda (baking soda)
2 cups (240 g/7 2/3 oz) gluten-free self-raising flour
1 teaspoon mixed spice
1/2 teaspoon ground cardamom
1/2 cup (115 g/3 2/3 oz) firmly packed brown sugar
2 eggs, lightly beaten
2 tablespoons olive oil
2 tablespoons poppy seeds

1 Preheat oven to 180°C (350°F/Gas 4). Grease and line a 24 cm x 12 cm (9 1/2 in x 5 in) loaf tin.
2 Put the dried fruit and water into a pan. Bring to the boil, then reduce the heat and simmer for 5 minutes or until nearly all the liquid has been absorbed. Remove from the heat and stir in the bicarbonate of soda.
3 Sift the flour, mixed spice and cardamom into a bowl, stir in the sugar and make a well in the center. Whisk together the eggs, oil and the cooled fruit mixture. Pour into the well and mix to combine.
4 Spoon the mixture into the prepared tin and sprinkle with the poppy seeds. Bake for 50 minutes or until a skewer comes out clean when inserted into the center. Allow to cool for 5 minutes before turning out on a wire rack to cool completely. Serves 10

per serve | fat 6.3 g | saturated fat 1 g | protein 6.3 g | carbohydrate 68.9 g | fibre 7.6 g | cholesterol 38 mg | energy 1467 kJ (349 Cal) | gi 64 ◆ med

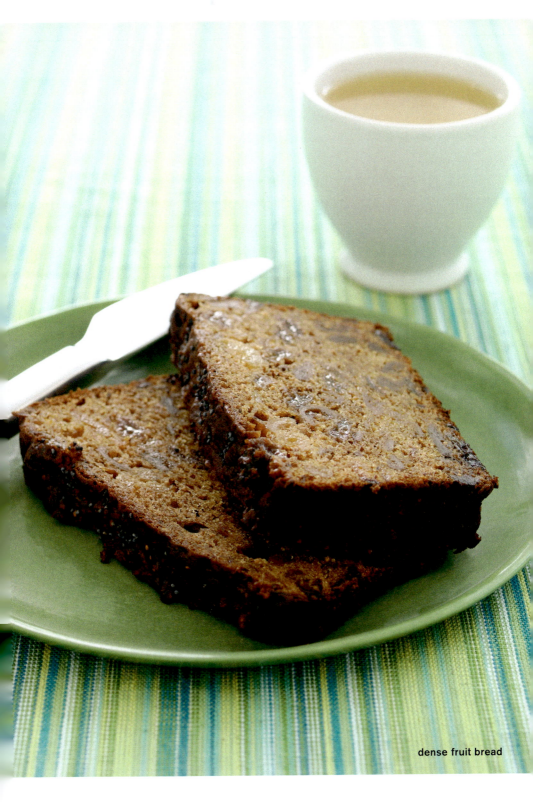
dense fruit bread

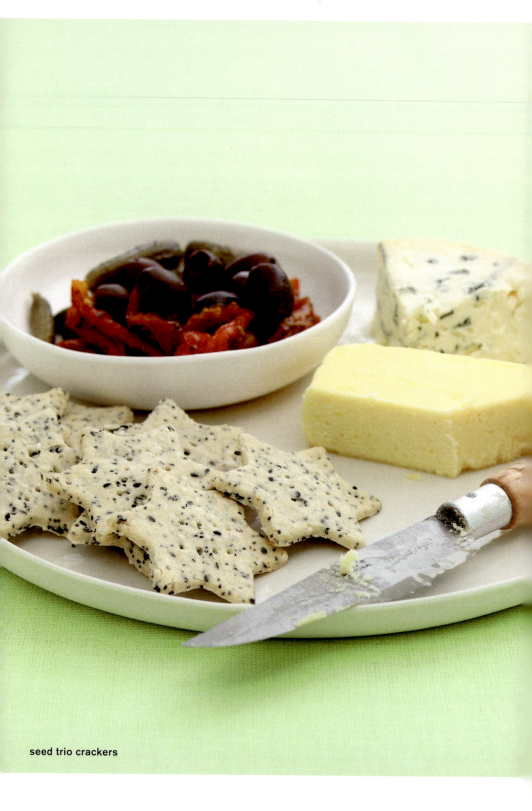
seed trio crackers

SEED TRIO CRACKERS

1 Preheat oven to 180°C (350°F/Gas 4). Line 2 baking trays with baking paper.
2 Sift the flour, baking powder and salt into a bowl and stir in the seeds. Rub in the butter or margarine until the mixture resembles fine breadcrumbs. Make a well in the center.
3 Gradually pour the water into the well and stir into the dry ingredients using a flat-bladed knife. Mix until the dough comes together, then gather into a ball.
4 Roll out half the dough between 2 sheets of baking paper until it is 2 mm (1/8 in) thick. Cut shapes from the dough using a star-shaped or round cutter. Repeat with the remaining dough. Put the shapes onto the prepared trays and prick all over with a fork. Bake for 20-25 minutes or until crisp. Transfer to a wire rack and leave to cool completely. Store in an airtight container for up to 5 days. Makes 30

per cracker | fat 2.9 g | saturated fat 0.8 g | protein 1.2 g | carbohydrate 5.7 g | fibre 0.8 g | cholesterol 3 mg | energy 229 kJ (55 Cal) | gi 55 ▼ low

- 2 cups (240 g/7 2/3 oz) gluten-free all-purpose flour pre mix
- 1 teaspoon gluten-free baking powder
- 1/2 teaspoon salt
- 2 tablespoons poppy seeds
- 2 tablespoons sesame seeds
- 2 tablespoons black sesame seeds
- 60 g (2 oz) butter or reduced-fat margarine, chopped
- 1/2 cup (125 ml/4 fl oz) iced water

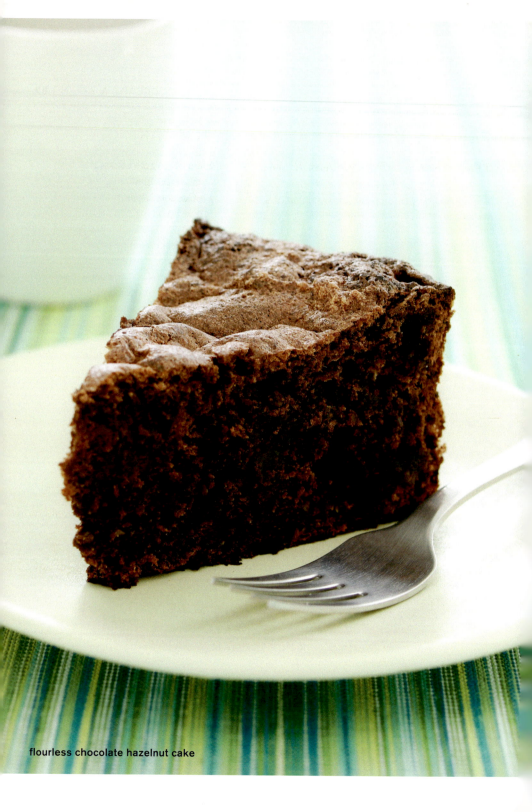

flourless chocolate hazelnut cake

FLOURLESS CHOCOLATE HAZELNUT CAKE

1 Preheat oven to 180°C (350°F/Gas 4). Line a 20 cm (8 in) spring form tin with baking paper.
2 Put the chocolate and milk into a heatproof bowl over a pan of simmering water. Do not let the base of the bowl touch the water. Stir over medium heat until the chocolate has melted. Set aside to cool slightly.
3 Put the chocolate mixture, hazelnut meal, sugar and egg yolks into a bowl and mix to combine.
4 Whisk the egg whites in a clean, dry bowl until stiff peaks form. Fold the egg whites into the chocolate mixture and spoon into the prepared tin. Bake for 45 minutes or until firm. Allow to cool in the tin for 5 minutes. Serve with fresh berries. Serves 8

per serve | fat 22.7 g | saturated fat 10.4 g | protein 8.4 g | carbohydrate 34.6 g | fibre 3 g | cholesterol 142 mg | energy 1559 kJ (371 Cal) | gi 50 ▼ low

- 250 g (8 oz) dark cooking chocolate, chopped
- 2 tablespoons milk
- 120 g (4 oz) hazelnut meal
- ½ cup (125 g/4 oz) caster sugar
- 6 eggs, separated

JAM DROPS

1 Preheat oven to 180°C (350°F/Gas 4). Line 2 baking trays with baking paper.
2 Beat the butter or margarine and sugar until light and creamy. Add the milk and vanilla and beat until combined. Add the sifted flour, rice cereal and custard powder and mix to form a soft dough.
3 Roll heaped teaspoons of the mixture into balls and place on the prepared trays. Gently flatten each ball and make an indentation in the center using the end of a wooden spoon.
4 Fill each hole with a little jam. Bake for 15 minutes or until golden. Allow to cool slightly on the trays before transferring to a wire rack to cool completely. Makes 20

per jam drop | fat 3.1 g | saturated fat 1.3 g | protein 0.5 g | carbohydrate 13.3 g | fibre 0.3 g | cholesterol 5 mg | energy 345 kJ (82 Cal) | gi 60 ◆ med

- 80 g (2⅔ oz) butter or reduced-fat margarine, softened
- ⅓ cup (90 g/3 oz) caster sugar
- 2 tablespoons milk
- ½ teaspoon vanilla essence
- ½ cup (60 g/2 oz) gluten-free all-purpose flour pre mix
- ¾ cup (45 g/1½ oz) baby rice cereal
- ⅓ cup (40 g/1⅓ oz) gluten-free custard powder
- ⅓ cup (100 g/3⅓ oz) raspberry jam

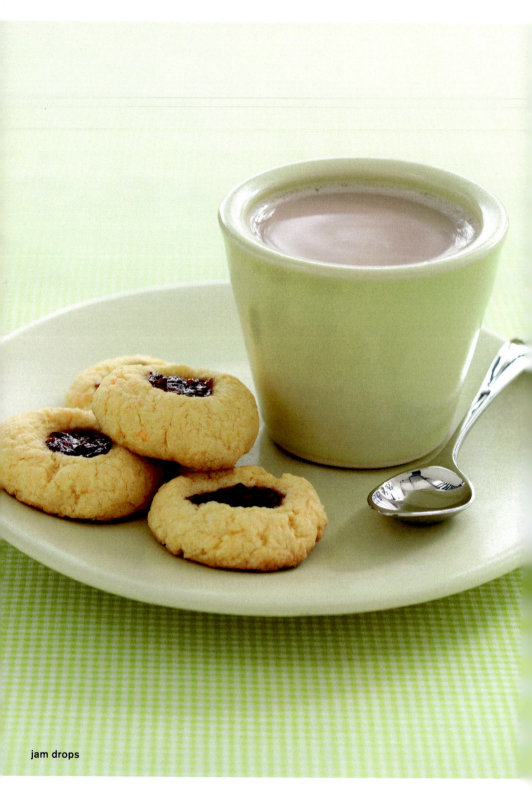
jam drops

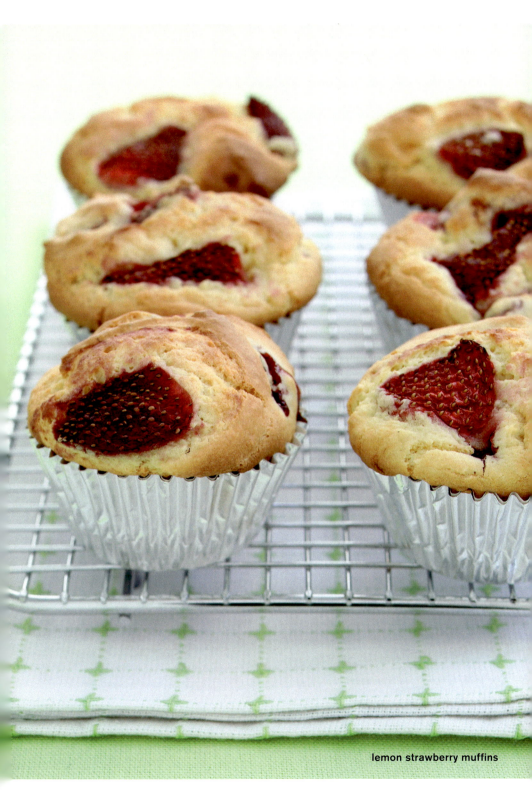
lemon strawberry muffins

LEMON STRAWBERRY MUFFINS

300 g (10 oz) strawberries, hulled
2½ cups (300 g/10 oz) gluten-free self-raising flour
⅔ cup (170 g/5⅔ oz) caster sugar
½ cup (30 g/1 oz) baby rice cereal
3 teaspoons lemon zest
1½ cups (375 ml/12 fl oz) skim or no-fat milk
2 eggs, lightly beaten
2 tablespoons vegetable oil

1 Preheat oven to 200°C (400°F/Gas 6). Line a 12 x ⅓ cup (80 ml/2⅔ fl oz) capacity muffin pan with muffin cases.
2 Roughly chop half the strawberries. Cut the remaining strawberries in half and set aside.
3 Sift the flour into a bowl, stir in the sugar, rice cereal, chopped strawberries and lemon zest and make a well in the center. Whisk together the milk, eggs and oil, pour into the well and gently mix with a metal spoon until the ingredients are just combined.
4 Divide the batter among the muffin cases. Press the reserved strawberries into the tops of the muffins. Bake for 15-20 minutes or until the muffins are golden and risen. Turn out on a wire rack to cool. Makes 12
per muffin | fat 4.3 g | saturated fat 0.7 g | protein 5.3 g | carbohydrate 35.7 g | fibre 1.6 g | cholesterol 32 mg | energy 854 kJ (203 Cal) | gi 59 ◆ med

ANZAC COOKIES

1½ cups (180 g/6 oz) gluten-free all-purpose flour pre mix
⅔ cup (170 g/5⅔ oz) caster sugar
¾ cup (60 g/2 oz) desiccated coconut
100 g (3⅓ oz) butter or reduced-fat margarine
¼ cup (60 ml/2 fl oz) water
¼ cup (60 ml/2 fl oz) golden syrup
1 cup (55 g/1⅔ oz) rice flakes with psyllium
½ teaspoon bicarbonate of soda (baking soda)

1 Preheat oven to 180°C (350°F/Gas 4). Line 2 baking trays with baking paper.
2 Sift the flour into a bowl, stir in the sugar and coconut and make a well in the center.
3 Put the butter or margarine, water, golden syrup and rice flakes into a pan and cook over low heat until melted and smooth. Set aside for 10 minutes.
4 Return the pan to the heat and cook for 5 minutes. Remove from the heat and stir in the bicarbonate of soda. Pour into the dry ingredients and mix to combine.
5 Drop tablespoons of mixture onto the prepared trays and flatten slightly with a fork. Bake for 20 minutes or until golden. Transfer to a wire rack to cool. Makes 26
per cookie | fat 4.5 g | saturated fat 2.5 g | protein 0.9 g | carbohydrate 15.7 g | fibre 1 g | cholesterol 5 mg | energy 447 kJ (106 Cal) | gi 57 ◆ med

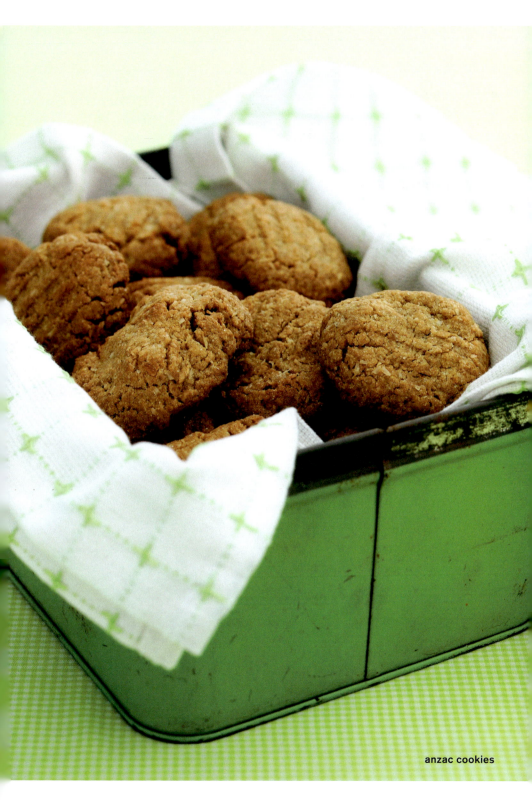
anzac cookies

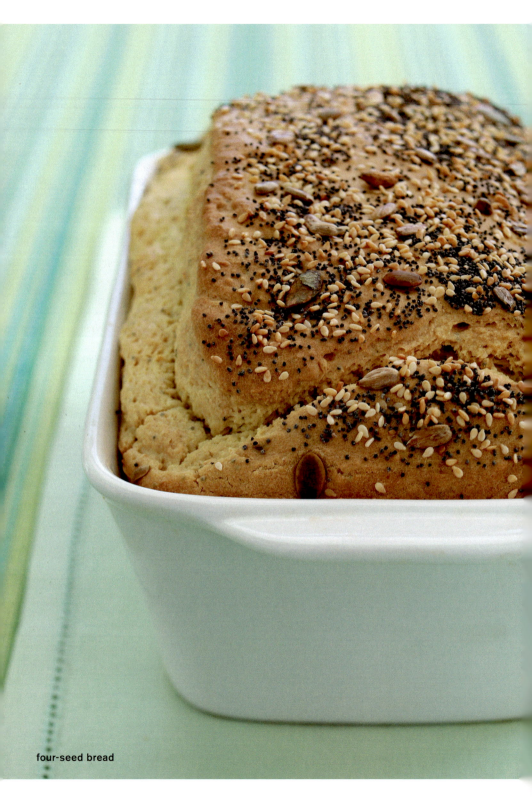

four-seed bread

FOUR-SEED BREAD

1 Preheat oven to 200°C (400°F/Gas 6). Lightly grease an ovenproof ceramic or glass loaf dish or 2 small loaf tins.
2 Sift the loaf mix, flour, salt and sugar into a bowl. Stir in the dried yeast, tartaric or citric acid and 3 tablespoons of the seeds. Make a well in the center.
3 Whisk together the eggs, water and oil, pour into the well and stir to combine. Mix well with electric beaters for 5 minutes.
4 Spoon the mixture into the prepared dish, cover with lightly oiled plastic wrap and set aside to rise in a warm place for 45 minutes.
5 Brush the loaf with a little water and sprinkle with the remaining seeds. Bake for 40 minutes or until the loaf has risen and is golden. Serves 10

per serve | fat 17 g | saturated fat 2.4 g | protein 7.2 g | carbohydrate 35.1 g | fibre 3.6 g | cholesterol 56 mg | energy 1371 kJ (327 Cal) | gi 57 ◆ med

* You may substitute the loaf mix with extra gluten-free all-purpose flour pre mix if preferred.

- 2 cups (240 g/7$^{2}/_{3}$ oz) gluten-free yeast-free loaf mix*
- 2 cups (240 g/7$^{2}/_{3}$ oz) gluten-free all-purpose flour pre mix
- ½ teaspoon salt
- 1 teaspoon sugar
- 2 teaspoons dried yeast
- ¼ teaspoon tartaric or citric acid
- 4 tablespoons mixed seeds (sunflower seeds, sesame seeds, pepitas, poppy seeds)
- 3 eggs, lightly beaten
- 2 cups (500 ml/16 fl oz) warm water
- ½ cup (125 ml/4 fl oz) olive oil

INDEX

anzac cookies 90
banana bread, coconut 79
beans, texas-style 10
beef noodle stir fry 35
beef yakitori 48
blueberries, crepes with 61
bolognese bake, polenta 42
bread, coconut banana 79
bread, dense fruit 82
bread, four-seed 93
bread rolls 77
caesar salad, chicken 45
cake, carrot 71
cake, flourless chocolate hazelnut 87
cake, middle eastern orange & almond 57
caramelised onion & fetta quiche 32
carrot cake 71
cheese, tomato & bacon corn bread 74
cheesecake, white chocolate raspberry 58
chicken caesar salad 45
chicken drumsticks, indian 38
chicken wraps, sweet chilli 35
chocolate hazelnut cake, flourless 87
chunky fruit yoghurts 18
coconut banana bread 79
coffee hazelnut chews 82
cookies, anzac 90
cookies, flourless fruit & nut 74
cookies & ice cream 61
corn bread, cheese, tomato & bacon 74
corn fritters with rocket & parmesan 13

crepes with blueberries 61
crepes, spinach & ricotta buckwheat 25
crumble, rhubarb 54
crunchy polenta fish & chips 27
crunchy raspberry rice pudding 67
date & polenta puddings, sticky 64
dense fruit bread 82
fish & chips, crunchy polenta 27
flourless chocolate hazelnut cake 87
flourless fruit & nut cookies 74
four-seed bread 93
frittatas, spinach, tomato & fetta pasta 27
fruit bread, dense 82
fruit yoghurts, chunky 18
gnocchi salad 22
granita, passionfruit & pineapple 64
ham, egg & tomato quesadillas 15
home-made muesli 10
ice cream, cookies & 61
indian chicken drumsticks 38
indian vegetable fritters 48
jam drops 87
lemon strawberry muffins 90
mango coconut sago pudding 54
meatloaf, thai 30
middle eastern orange & almond cake 57
muesli, home-made 10
muffins, lemon strawberry 90
mushroom, bacon & pea risotto 51
noodle stir fry, beef 35
orange & almond cake, middle eastern 57
pancakes, ricotta buckwheat 15
parmesan & pepper shortbread 79

passionfruit & pineapple granita 64
pizzas, tomato, olive & bocconcini 41
polenta bolognese bake 42
polenta porridge 18
porridge, polenta 18
prawn rice paper rolls 30
quesadillas, ham, egg & tomato 15
quiche, caramelised onion & fetta 32
raspberry rice pudding, crunchy 67
rhubarb crumble 54
rice pudding, crunchy raspberry 67
ricotta buckwheat pancakes 15
risotto, mushroom, bacon & pea 51
sago pudding, mango coconut 54
salmon patties, sweet potato & 45
seed trio crackers 85
shortbread, parmesan & pepper 79
souffles, vanilla & saffron rice 68
spicy tuna tacos 22
spinach & ricotta buckwheat crepes 25
spinach, tomato & fetta pasta frittatas 27
sticky date & polenta puddings 64
stir fry, beef noodle 35
sweet chilli chicken wraps 35
sweet potato & salmon patties 45
tacos, spicy tuna 22
texas-style beans 10
thai meatloaf 30
tomato, olive & bocconcini pizzas 41
tuna tacos, spicy 22
vanilla & saffron rice souffles 68
vegetable fritters, indian 48
vegetable millet cakes 38
white chocolate raspberry cheesecake 58
yoghurts, chunky fruit 18

95 ACKNOWLEDGEMENTS

Publisher Jody Vassallo
General manager Claire Connolly
Recipes & styling Jody Vassallo
Photographer Ben Dearnley
Home economist Penelope Grieve
Recipe testing Cilah Ralph
Props stylists Melissa Singer, Trish Hegarty
Designer Annette Fitzgerald
Editor Justine Harding
Consultant dietitian Dr Susanna Holt
Introduction Kim Faulkner-Hogg

STYLING CREDITS:
Bayswiss (02) 9411 4344
Bison Homewares (02) 6284 2334
Country Road (02) 9960 4633
Design Mode International (02) 9998 8200
Mud Australia (02) 9518 0220
Orrefors Kosta Boda (02) 9415 4912
Wheel & Barrow (02) 9938 4555
Appliances used in this book provided by Sunbeam Corporation Limited.
© **Recipes** Jody Vassallo 2003
© **Photography** Ben Dearnley
© **Series design** Fortiori Publishing

Print management Steve Allan, Web Production

PUBLISHED BY FORTIORI PUBLISHING:
PO Box 126 Nunawading BC
Victoria 3110 Australia
Phone: 61 3 9872 3855
Fax: 61 3 9872 5454
salesenquiries@fortiori.com.au
www.fortiori.com.au
order direct on (03) 9872 3855

Printed by McPherson's Printing Group.
Printed in Australia.

ISBN 0 9581609 5 3

This publication is copyright. No part may be reproduced, stored in a retrieval system or transmitted in any form or by any means whether electronic, mechanical, photocopied, recorded or otherwise without the prior written permission of the publisher. Australian distribution to newsagents and supermarkets by Gordon and Gotch Ltd, 68 Kingsgrove Road, Belmore, NSW 2192.

DISCLAIMER: The nutritional information listed under each recipe does not include the nutrient content of garnishes or any accompaniments not listed in specific quantities in the ingredient list. The nutritional information for each recipe is an estimate only, and may vary depending on the brand of ingredients used, and due to natural biological variations in the composition of natural foods such as meat, fish, fruit and vegetables. The nutritional information was calculated by a qualified dietitian using FoodWorks dietary analysis software (Professional Version 3.10, Xyris Software Pty Ltd, Highgate Hill, Queensland, Australia) based on the Australian food composition tables and food manufacturers' data. Where not specified, ingredients are analysed as average or medium. All recipes were analysed using 59 g eggs.

The GI values listed for each recipe are estimates only and were calculated by an experienced dietitian using published GI values for each of the carbohydrate-containing ingredients in the recipe. If an ingredient didn't have a published GI value, the GI value of the most similar foodstuff was used as a substitute. For this reason, and the fact that food preparation and cooking methods can affect a food's GI value, it is not possible to estimate the GI value of a recipe exactly, although it's likely that the recipe's estimated GI category (low, medium or high) will be correct. People with diabetes should measure their own blood glucose responses to the recipes in order to find the meals that give them the lowest blood glucose responses.

IMPORTANT: Those who might suffer particularly adverse effects from salmonella food poisoning (the elderly, pregnant women, young children and those with immune system problems) should consult their general practitioner about consuming raw or undercooked eggs.

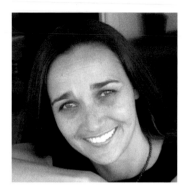

Producing a cookbook can be an arduous process; fortunately, for me it is a truly pleasurable experience that is enriched by the wonderful team of experienced professionals I work alongside. My partners **Claire, Helen and Peter** provide me with a constant source of encouragement, creative input and positive feedback, and, most importantly, they are responsible for selling the beautiful books I make. **Justine Harding**, my angel in editing chair, makes sure I stay on schedule and her fine-tooth comb ensures the books are as accurate as any cookbook could possibly be. **Annette Fitzgerald**, my gifted designer, lays out the pages and creates the overall look of the book. **Ben Dearnley**, photographer extraordinaire, captures the essence of my food in a way that still amazes me - his ability to make something so simple look simply sumptuous is a God-given gift. **Penel Grieve**, my dear friend and amazingly talented kitchen wizardess, prepares each recipe with the most essential ingredient - a little pinch of her own pure, loving spirit. **Susanna Holt**, woman of health, then analyses each recipe with her ever-watchful professional eye. **Melissa Singer**, style princess, gathers the gorgeous fabrics that make each book truly outstanding. **Trish Hegarty** sources the beautiful props. **Scott Bradford** then ensures each pic looks as good as it possibly can on paper.

My loving friends and family continue to allow me to subject them to weeks of tasting, providing me with constructive, honest criticism that is truly invaluable. Earth mother **Judy Clarke** sat with me for hours helping me formulate what people with coeliac disease would want in a cookbook, something only she could do after having spent years working in a health-food store. My calm, collected flatmate **Col**, who has an insatiable appetite for leftovers, allows me to transform our home into a photographic studio with props strewn from one end to the other. **Pride Joy**, my precious darling dog daughter, eats my favourite footwear, traumatises small white dogs with owners much larger than me and reminds me that there is more to life than hanging out in the kitchen.

This book, however, would not have been possible without **Di Boyle** - the gluten free expert. Di, thank you so much for sharing your expert knowledge unconditionally. Your enthusiasm for helping me understand the intricacies of gluten-free baking truly touched my heart. I could never have created the quiche, carrot cake, cheesecake or Anzacs without your secret ingredient. Thank you to **Kim Faulkner-Hogg** for writing the introduction and for your advice on what people with coeliac disease eat. And finally, to all the people out there who suffer from coeliac disease... this is for you. I hope your tummies enjoy these recipes as much as mine did. **Happy cooking!**